"YOU ARE GORGEOUS . . .
you deserve satisfaction and laughter in your life. You deserve
pleasure. You deserve love. I can tell you this a thousand times,
but you won't believe me until you experience it yourself. You
won't believe me until you begin acting as if you already believe
it. . . .

"Learning about your hunger, tasting a raisin as if it were the
first you ever ate, stopping when you are satisfied, it's all part
of waking up to being alive. . . ."

—Geneen Roth

By teaching you to trust your body and yourself . . . to put aside
self-judgment . . . to conquer the obsession with food and
dieting, this unique and practical workbook will help you to find
out what it is you're really hungering for. From there, breaking
free is only a matter of time.

WHY WEIGHT?

GENEEN ROTH is a writer and a teacher who has gained inter-
national prominence through her work in the field of eating
disorders. She is the founder of the Breaking Free workshops,
which she has conducted nationwide since 1979. She is also the
author of *Feeding the Hungry Heart, Breaking Free from Compulsive
Eating,* and *When Food Is Love.* A frequent guest on television and
radio programs, she has written for and been featured in *Time,
Ms., New Woman, Family Circle,* and *Cosmopolitan.* Her poetry and
short stories have been published in numerous anthologies.
Born in New York City, she now lives in northern California.

D0950577

Other books by Geneen Roth:

FEEDING THE HUNGRY HEART
BREAKING FREE FROM COMPULSIVE EATING

WHY WEIGHT?

A GUIDE TO
ENDING
COMPULSIVE EATING

GENEEN ROTH

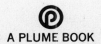

A PLUME BOOK

To Peg Parkinson, my editor and friend,
without whom my writing would have remained in
my journals
and my dreams would have remained only dreams.

PLUME
Published by the Penguin Group
Penguin Books USA Inc., 375 Hudson Street, New York, New York
10014, U.S.A.
Penguin Books Ltd, 27 Wrights Lane, London W8 5TZ, England
Penguin Books Australia Ltd, Ringwood, Victoria, Australia
Penguin Books Canada Ltd, 2801 John Street, Markham, Ontario, Canada
L3R 1B4
Penguin Books (N.Z.) Ltd, 182-190 Wairau Road, Auckland 10, New Zealand

Penguin Books Ltd, Registered Offices: Harmondsworth, Middlesex, England

Published by Plume, an imprint of New American Library, a division of
Penguin Books USA Inc.

BOOKS ARE AVAILABLE AT QUANTITY DISCOUNTS WHEN USED TO PROMOTE
PRODUCTS OR SERVICES. FOR INFORMATION PLEASE WRITE TO PREMIUM
MARKETING DIVISION, PENGUIN BOOKS USA INC. 375 HUDSON STREET,
NEW YORK, NEW YORK 10014.

PUBLISHER'S NOTE

The ideas, procedures, and suggestions contained in this book are not intended
as a substitute for consulting with your physician. All matters regarding your
health require medical supervision.

 REGISTERED TRADEMARK—MARCA REGISTRADA

Library of Congress Cataloging-in-Publication Data

Roth, Geneen.
    Why weight? : a guide to ending compulsive eating/Geneen Roth.
        p.   cm.
    ISBN 0-452-26254-2
    1. Compulsive eating—Popular works.   I. Title.
RC552.C65R67   1989
616.85′2—dc19   88-35324
                                                                        CIP

Designed by A. K. Amann

First Printing, June, 1989

6   7   8   9   10   11   12   13

PRINTED IN THE UNITED STATES OF AMERICA

CONTENTS

Acknowledgments

Without Sara Friedlander, this book would not have been written. She provided enthusiasm when I had none, ideas when I drew a blank, matzoh balls when I needed food, and unflagging devotion to this project, to my well-being, and to our work together. Sprawled beside me at 8 a.m. or 11 p.m., she edited my writing, drew charts, suggested exercises, and rushed with me to the vet when we thought Blanche had cactus needles caught in his nose. This book is as much Sara's as it is mine.

Jace Schinderman provided the structure for the book. She was the first person in the book chain, sending outlines and exercises to me by Federal Express and putting her life on hold as she absorbed my work and became an expert in curing compulsive eating. For eighteen years, she has been there whenever I have needed her, and this time was no exception.

I am deeply grateful to the participants of the Breaking Free workshops who continue to inspire me with their courage and their vulnerability. And to everyone who has written to me since the publication of *Breaking Free From Compulsive Eating*, telling me their own stories and asking for help. This book is for them, for you.

I would also like to thank: Angela Miller for finding the way out; Nancy Wechsler for her keen mind and sympathetic soul; Maureen Nemeth for her loyalty and competence; Becky Luening for the speed and sensitivity she brings to her work; Judith Lateer for a fine beginning; Jane Mycue and Judith Scott for taking such good care of Blanche and me; and Elaine Koster for making it clear that my writing was worth waiting for.

Finally, I want to thank Matt Weinstein for so much of everything, but, this time in particular, for knowing when to laugh and when to take me seriously, and for teaching me to do the same.

Introduction

I was a compulsive eater for seventeen years. I went on every diet I heard of or read about: the prunes-and-meatball diet, the one-hot-fudge-sundae-a-day diet, the applesauce-and-chicken-wing diet, Stillman's, Atkin's, and Weight Watchers. I lost weight on all of them—usually I spent three weeks losing ten pounds and four days gaining it back. But gaining the weight back (often with a bonus of two or three pounds) wasn't the worst part. The worst part was how much I suffered through all of it. There were many times when I awoke at three in the morning, sweating and breathless, having dreamed of slicing off pieces of my thighs, my arms, even portions of my face. I felt that mutilating myself would not hurt more than having thunderous thighs, upper arms that flapped, and cheeks that were as round and pasty as a Chinese pork bun.

I stopped dieting nine years ago on a day that I remember well: I took the rusty old postage scales that I had been using to weigh each ounce of food I ate and I threw them into the garbage. I tore up my diet charts and burned them in my bathtub. Then, I told myself I could eat whatever I wanted whenever I was hungry.

I was terrified.

The determination not to diet was the most frightening decision I had ever made. Anyone who has ever believed that if she listened to her hunger she would destroy herself, knows the extent of that pervasive and very real fear.

I stopped dieting because the pain of what I was doing to myself was greater than the fear of being fat for the rest of my life. I stopped dieting because I was suicidal—the struggle with my weight had become a matter of life and death. I planned ways to kill myself: driving over the cliffs on Highway One;

swallowing a bottle of Clorox; slitting my wrists on the blue tile floor in the bathroom. I stopped dieting because not one diet worked and I realized that if I wanted to be certain of being fat for the rest of my life, the best way was *not* to stop dieting.

In time, and by following the guidelines described in this book, my body reached its natural weight. But being thinner is not the best part; the best part is living a life in which I am not obsessed about food. The best part is knowing that the answers are not outside me, in any prescribed diet. The answers are within me—in my head, my heart, my stomach. I can listen to myself; I will not destroy myself. When I am hungry, I can eat; when I need comfort, I can ask for it. The power and joy I feel now, compared with the helplessness and utter despair I felt for 17 years, is the best part. And it gets better and better.

In the years since I wrote *Feeding the Hungry Heart* and *Breaking Free*, I've received over ten thousand letters from people who are at different points upon the path of breaking free from compulsive eating. They thank me for the books and then they ask if I can help them. Can I tell them about the Breaking Free workshops, can I please suggest a way out of their hellish worlds of eating, it is so dark in there. Please, Ms. Roth, please.

When I was an anorexic, I fasted for three weeks during the change of every season, telling myself that I was doing it for health reasons: to cleanse my liver and kidneys of stored toxins. I drank vegetable juice one week and diluted fruit juice the second week, and I fasted on water for the last week. After I broke the fast, I spent a week eating fruit. When the month was over, I weighed myself; I usually lost twenty pounds. Then my binge began: chocolate-covered donuts, sugar cookies the size of serving plates, whole pizzas, a dozen pieces of fried chicken at one sitting. In the middle of one of these after-a-fast binges, I wrote a frantic letter to the author of a book on fasting. I begged him for help. Please, Mr. Kulvinskas, please. His reply to me was short: Be kind to yourself, he advised, stop punishing yourself. I was grateful that he wrote back to me, but I had *no idea* how to be kind to myself. He might have been writing in Sanskrit, for all I knew of self-kindness.

When I answer letters, I, too, tell people to be kind to themselves. I tell them to listen to their hungers, to practice nourishing themselves in ways other than eating, to find support for themselves in something other than food. But they wouldn't be writing me if they knew how.

Why Weight? is a guide to being kind to yourself through each step of the journey of breaking free from compulsive eating. The book is written in workbook form so that you have the space actually to *do*—not just think about doing—the exercises. You cannot *think* your way out of an obsession with food. You must make a commitment. You must take time. You must feel that the pain of what you are doing to yourself with food is greater than the fear of trusting yourself. You must believe that the serenity and profound joy of living a life free of the obsession with food is stronger than the fear of what will happen when you begin.

My intent in writing this workbook is to provide you with both the concrete structure that you can use to change the way you eat and the tools that will teach you to care for yourself in other ways. The exercises were developed from the physical and emotional struggles and victories of my own experience as well as those of participants in the Breaking Free workshops that I lead.

Why Weight? is filled with ideas, exercises and suggestions. You may find some of them difficult, scary, or time-consuming, or maybe just different enough so that you don't want to do them. That's understandable; notice your reluctance gently and *then* do the exercises. Change is the result of taking risks, of going a step beyond what is comfortable. Reluctance to do an exercise may in fact indicate that the topic of that exercise, and your fears about doing it, need special attention.

Work at your own pace. Spend time each day answering the questions, practicing the exercises. Your time will not be wasted; you *will* begin to notice a difference in yourself.

Many people who hear that I do not believe in dieting protest that they need to go on a diet first, lose ten pounds, and *then* begin following my guidelines. I understand how frightening it can be, suddenly to be told to listen to your body and trust its wisdom after a lifetime of being told what and when to eat. But I also know that you can spend the next ten years dieting so that you will be ready to stop dieting.

There is nothing to wait for.

The process you will go through as you do the exercises in the book—the feeling of exhilaration, the wonder at the complex and ultimately reliable body of yours, the fear of eating everything that isn't moving and the intense satisfaction when you don't—is the goal. The goal is not to lose ten or twenty or a hundred pounds; the goal is to live more fully, love more deeply. To be who you know you can be when you are not diminishing yourself by the obsession with food: that's the best part.

—Geneen Roth
Santa Cruz, California

CHAPTER 1

Compulsion and Awareness

We become compulsive for very good reasons. We're not here *not to be here*. We're not here to rip ourselves apart. We're not here to make ourselves miserable. When it looks as if that's what we're doing—when, by our eating, it looks as if we are trying to destroy ourselves—it's time to look deeper. It's time to look again. It's time to piece together some of the things that don't seem to make sense and acknowledge that, in fact, they really *do* make sense.

We begin simply and gently: by becoming aware of what we are doing and how we are trying to care for ourselves. Remember that compulsive eating is *always* an attempt to care for yourself. Many people have a hard time believing that. We want to lose weight so badly, we want to be done with problems about food immediately (because we've already spent too many years worrying, dieting, bingeing), that it's a tremendous leap of faith for us to believe that our eating serves a valuable purpose in our lives. To stop eating compulsively, we must take the time to examine what that purpose is.

You cannot take away a compulsion unless you replace it with something else. You cannot stop eating compulsively unless you acknowledge the needs it is serving and find new and more satisfying ways to fill those needs.

The first step, then, is to become aware of what you are doing and how it is serving you.

Exercise 1: Who Am I?

Take time now to introduce yourself to yourself. Next to the introduction below, write down the name you want to be known by. Then, ten times repeated, say the phrase "I am . . ." and complete the sentence with a description of yourself. The sentence can be short or long, abstract or concrete. You can do this exercise quickly or slowly.

INTRODUCTION OF_____

I am <u>a woman.</u>

I am <u>a prisoner in my body.</u>

I am <u>thirty-five years old.</u>

I am <u>funny.</u>

I am _____

I am _____

I am _____

I am _____

I am _____

I am _____

I am _____

I am _____

I am _____

I am _____

Take a ten-minute break and look back over the list you made. Do you see things that surprise you? Any themes running through them? As you use this workbook, you may want to return to this page and reread it. Or you may want to rewrite the "I am . . ." to see how you are feeling about yourself on a particular day.

Exercise 2: Life Without Compulsive Eating

Most of us believe that if we didn't have conflicts about food our lives would be wonderful. We would be happy, beautiful, free. But the truth is that compulsive eating takes up a huge amount of our time—thinking about it, planning binges, worrying about our bodies, strategizing about how different life will be when we are thin. Without compulsive eating, our lives really would be drastically different.

What *would* your life be like if you were thin? If you were to live with no conflicts about food, how would the way you live and the quality of your days be different?

Complete the sentence:
If I didn't have conflicts about food . . .

EXAMPLES:
1) I would have much more energy than I do now.
2) My friends would wonder how I did it and feel threatened by me.

I would _____

_____

My life would _____

_____

My friends would _____

_____

My family would _____

_____

My days would _____

_____

My dreams in life would _____

_____

Exercise 3: The Fat Me

List the qualities you associate with being fat. Describe the fat you. Who are you? What do you do? How do you feel? Be specific about the clothes you wear, the things you say, the work you do. Are you strong? Fragile? Sensitive? Outgoing? Concerned with other people's feelings?

The Fat Me is:

EXAMPLES:
1) plodding
2) awkward
3) safe

_____

_____

_____

_____

_____

_____

_____

_____

The Fat Me wears clothes that are:

EXAMPLES:
1) shapeless
2) dark

_____

_____

_____

_____

When I am at a party, the Fat Me:

_____

_____

_____

_____

When I am alone, the Fat Me:

_____

_____

_____

_____

The Fat Me likes:

_____

_____

_____

_____

Exercise 4: Why Weight?

Complete the following list:

Being fat enables me to:

EXAMPLES:
1) have excuses for not quitting my job.
2) eat whatever I want.
3) know who likes me for my body and who likes me for myself.

_____

_____

_____

_____

Exercise 5: The Thin Me

List the qualities you associate with being thin. Describe the thin you. This you is most assuredly different from the fat you in what you say, do, wear. Who *is* this you?

The Thin Me is:
1) sexy.
2) outgoing.

_____

_____

_____

_____

_____

The Thin Me wears clothes that are:

_____

_____

_____

_____

_____

When I am at a party, the Thin Me:

_____

_____

_____

_____

When I am alone, the Thin Me:

_____

_____

_____

_____

The Thin Me deserves:

_____

_____

_____

_____

_____

Exercise 6: The No's of Being Thin

Although we might not recognize this reality, being thin can carry a burden of its own. For instance, if I feel that when I am thin I must be vivacious and socially active, *and* I am a solitary human being by nature, I am not going to want to get thin. I will unconsciously block myself from achieving my goal—even while staying frustrated and impatient that I can't reach it. It is therefore important for us to become aware of what we believe about being thin, and most especially, what those things are that are important for us to do, that we don't believe we will be able to go on doing if we get thin.

Complete this list.

Being thin means I can't:
1) be insecure or quiet or afraid.
2) have another chocolate bar as long as I live.

_____

_____

_____

_____

_____

Do you surprise yourself with your completions of these statements?
   Notice how your weight and size speak for you, how they express who you are and how you feel.

Exercise 7: Weight History

If we look back on our lives and the times we have gained or lost significant amounts of weight, we will probably notice a connection among our outer circumstances, our emotions, and the way we used food. When we identify this connection, we can make better choices about expressing conflicts and feelings in a direct way, with words and actions, rather than with our bodies.

Beginning with the first time you can remember losing and/or gaining a significant amount of weight, write down the corresponding events that were taking place in your life and the feelings that you had about them.

Weight Loss/Gain	Events	Feelings
Lost 15 pounds	I was 11; I realized my parents were unhappy.	Scared, lonely
Gained 10 pounds	Sheldon died.	Desperate, miserable

Weight Loss/Gain	Events	Feelings

Weight Loss/Gain	Events	Feelings

Exercise 8: What Am I Waiting for?

Most compulsive eaters are waiting until they have the "right" body to begin living the kind of life they want to live. You don't have to wait. You deserve to have what you want now. *Being thin* does not suddenly make you worthy of a job you like, relationships that are meaningful, clothes that you find attractive. *Your decision* that you are worthy is what makes you worthy.

What are you waiting to get thin to do?

Complete the following list.
I am waiting to get thin so I can:
1) go to my high school reunion and not be ashamed of myself.
2) be in a relationship.
3) make love with the lights on.

_____

_____

_____

_____

_____

_____

_____

_____

_____

Read over the list. Pick two things on it that you can begin doing this week. Make a commitment to yourself to do them on specific days. You'll find that when you begin *acting as if* you deserve to treat yourself, and to be treated, with respect and kindness, you will slowly begin believing that you do.

Complete the sentence:
This week I will:

1) _____

2) _____

Exercise 9: A Dialogue with Fat

In my struggle with weight and my attempts to discover how it was serving me, I wrote a dialogue with my fat, asking it how it was trying to help me and telling it how I felt about its being such a big part of my life. That dialogue was a turning point for me because I realized, maybe for the first time, that no matter what I said or felt about my weight, it really was protecting me in a way that I did not believe I could protect myself. I realized that my fat was my friend, that I ate for very good reasons—and I began respecting myself for trying to take such good care of myself.

Allow at least one hour for your dialogue with your fat. If you do not feel fat, hold a dialogue with "compulsive eater," or whoever it is in you that you feel has the problems with food.

Begin by saying hello.

For example:
Me: Hello, Fat. Are you there?
Fat: I am always here.
Me: That's what the problem is. You are everywhere. You are ruining my life.
Fat: But I am not the one who lifts up the spoons and forks and puts the food into your mouth. You are.
Me: Stop trying to be so cute, Fat. You're the problem around here, not me. Why won't you go away?
Fat: Because you need me here. You think that if I weren't here, you wouldn't be able to . . .

Now it's your turn. Use the space below to write the dialogue.

Me:_____

_____

_____

_____

Fat:_____

_____

_____

_____

Me:_____

_____

_____

_____

Fat:_____

_____

_____

_____

Me:_____

_____

_____

_____

Me:_____

_____

_____

_____

Fat:_____

_____

_____

_____

Me:_____

_____

_____

_____

Fat:_____

_____

_____

_____

Me:_____

_____

_____

_____

_____

Me:_____

_____

_____

_____

Fat:_____

_____

_____

_____

Me:_____

_____

_____

_____

Fat:_____

_____

_____

_____

Me:_____

_____

_____

_____

CHAPTER 2
The Basics

When I was on a national TV show a few years ago, the interviewer began by asking me about my work. I told him that I wrote and led workshops for compulsive eaters. He said, "Could you tell me a little bit about your philosophy?"

So I said, "I believe that the basis of compulsive eating is emotional and that people really need to learn to *listen* to their hungers. It's important for them to eat when they're hungry, to stop when they've had enough, and to deal with the emotional conflicts they express by eating."

He said, "Is that it? Is that what you wrote a book about?"

"No, that's what I wrote two books about." He didn't believe what I was saying. He didn't believe that anyone could lose weight without going on a diet.

Although most of us are afraid that if we don't have a step-by-step program to tell us what, when, and how much to eat, we will never make any changes, I believe that the most important element in change is self-trust. The willingness to listen to the voice that wants to care for us, not destroy us.

If you have been following programs that tell you what and how much to eat, it may be overwhelming to be told that if you listen to your body, *it* will guide you in making healthy choices.

The Eating Guidelines are the basic structure of Breaking Free. They are not rules with which to punish yourself; they are suggestions that I found useful as I made a commitment to be conscious when I ate. After years of stolen eating, I needed a place to begin. The Guidelines helped me actually enjoy food

17

instead of making a mad dash for the refrigerator and eating all I could before I—or anyone—noticed what I was doing.

You may want to use the Guidelines as reference points for now. We will be working with each of them extensively in the chapters to come; read them over and take note of your reactions to them.

The Eating Guidelines

The Eating Guidelines are the core of the Breaking Free program. They are as follows:

1. Eat when you are hungry.
2. Eat sitting down in a calm environment. This does not include the car.
3. Eat without distractions. Distractions include radio, television, newspapers, books, intense or anxiety-producing conversations, and music.
4. Eat only what you want.
5. Eat until you are satisfied.
6. Eat (with the intention of being) in full view of others.
7. Eat with enjoyment, pleasure, and gusto.

Exercise 10: First Reactions

Which guidelines made you uncomfortable?

Number _____, because_____

_____

Number _____, because_____

_____

Number _____, because_____

_____

Which guidelines do you already practice?

Number _____; Number _____; Number _____

Which were completely new to you?

Number _____; Number _____; Number _____

Other Thoughts?

_____

_____

_____

_____

_____

_____

The Stages of Breaking Free

By watching myself carefully and by listening to the participants in workshops, I've developed what I think is a natural progression of stages that you go through as you follow the eating guidelines and explore the conflicts and feelings you use food to express and/or avoid. Keep in mind that there are no rigid timelines; everyone must go at her or his own pace. I offer this interpretation of the Stages of Breaking Free because many people find it reassuring to know that they are on a well-trodden path and are not alone.

Stage I: *Acknowledging That There Is a Problem,* that the problem is more complex than simply being overweight, and that dieting does not, and will never, resolve it.

Stage II: *Beginning/Rebelling Against the Years of Deprivation*

Physical Aspects:

- Eating mainly (what were previously) "forbidden" foods; eating all the time — not just when hungry and until satisfied.
- Learning what hunger, satisfaction, and fullness feel like.
- Learning what makes eating pleasurable (i.e., sitting, not reading or watching TV, eating slowly, etc.).
- Possibly gaining weight.

Emotional Aspects:

- Relief and exhilaration at not dieting.
- Panic and fear that this stage will go on forever, and that because this looks like a binge, breaking free is no different from bingeing.
- Sometimes there will be a feeling of hopelessness, a feeling that there is no end to compulsive eating.

Tips:
- Don't panic at the weight gain. It is *not* atypical, and it *is* a natural reaction to years of deprivation. You will *not* gain a hundred pounds.
- Throw away your scales, or paste your ideal weight on them.
- Try to distinguish between foods you think you want (because before you weren't allowed to have them) and foods you really *do* want in the present moment.

This stage will end. Do not go on another diet because you are afraid the stage will never end.

Stage III: *"The Middle" Nitty Gritty/Learning-to-Trust-and-Befriend -Yourself Stage*

Physical Aspects:
- Eating without guilt.
- No more bingeing.
- Weight stabilizes.
- Distinguishing foods you really like/want from those that were previously forbidden (they were hummers/beckoners).
- Ability to eat only a bite or two of chocolate.
- Foods other than sweets begin to taste good—you learn what nourishes you.
- You begin to have faith in body-wisdom as you see that you can eat what you want and not gain weight.
- You eat when you are hungry although, often, don't stop at just enough.

Emotional Aspects:
- The mind still wants more food than the body, which is a little difficult to accept.
- A lot of joy in realizing that after all these years, your body can still get hungry.
- A sense of power develops as you see that you can control food—it no longer controls you.

This is the hard-work stage: You can stop eating when you're not hungry, and the emotions that drove you to eat in the first place surface. If you are willing to work with yourself, you develop ways of dealing with your feelings other than using food. Some of these ways are:

• Keeping a journal.
• Being in therapy.
• Talking with friends about your feelings.
• Expressing your feelings as they arise.

You learn that food isn't all that's good or pleasurable about life. You learn many other ways of nourishing yourself:

• Taking walks, baths, naps.
• Reading.
• Going to movies.
• Meeting with friends.
• Getting massaged.
• Doing something you've always wanted to do.
• Writing.
• Dancing.

You begin to value things about yourself other than your body—and begin to realize that other people value you as well.

Your values about living change as you see that you can feel happy and satisfied without being thin; your inner life becomes important.

Tips:
• Weight loss might occur but it is not the predominant characteristic of this stage.
• What *is* predominant is the shift you make from viewing yourself as an out-of-control human being to one who can make choices that will nourish yourself.

This stage is the most difficult one because of all the feelings that arise, and it takes "an ocean of patience" and renewed commitment to the Breaking Free process. Remember that this is a *stage*, and that it will end.

The fear that often occurs in this stage is that if you deal with your compulsive eating and lose weight, you will no longer have an excuse (i.e, your fat) on which to blame all your "failures"— and that's true! But on the other hand, you'll have more available energy. You'll feel better about yourself, and you won't need an excuse.

Stage IV: *The Joys of Breaking Free*

Physical Aspects:

- Weight loss occurs—slowly!
- You eat what you want, stop when you're satisfied.
- What you want has drastically changed from Stage II. What you want now are usually nourishing foods with occasional or small bites of sweets instead of large amounts of sweets and occasional scrambled eggs.
- You enjoy your body. You *accept* your body, even though it is not perfect.
- Food becomes delightful, rather than a source of pain.
- When you're not hungry, you don't think about eating.
- You can go anywhere, have any kind of food in front of you, without going on a binge/eating compulsively.

Emotional Aspects:

- You ask for what you want as well as *eat* what you want.
- You feel better about yourself than you ever imagined you could feel. You are self-confident, self-trusting.
- This confidence and trust extend into many other areas of your life—your work, your relationships.

- Since your life is no longer revolving around food, you have more energy with which to *live*.
- You have many more skills with which to deal with problems.

Tips:
- Sometimes you, like anyone else, will overeat. But now you will not take it as a sign that you are a failure.
- Your weight will fluctuate by five to eight pounds from season to season. Sometimes you will want to eat more than you do at other times. That's okay—sometimes your body *needs* more food.

Exercise 11: Where Am I?

Some people are in Stage 1 and Stage 2 simultaneously; some people take a year to go through Stage 1 and Stage 2 and two months to go through Stage 3. *Wherever you are is absolutely fine.* And as long as it takes you to complete each stage is also absolutely fine. Judgment has no place in any part of Breaking Free.

I am in Stage __. The food issues I am dealing with in my life

right now are _____

and _____

Wherever you are in the stages, acknowledge yourself for the effort it's taken to get there.

The Eating Chart

Keeping an eating chart is like using a road map. If you don't know where you are, you cannot possibly find the way to your destination. Many of us (myself included) have strong feelings about keeping a chart. It reminds us of our dieting days, when we had to keep track of calories, carbohydrates, and how many carrots we ate in the morning. When I began eating consciously, however, I kept a chart every day for one year—I wrote down every bite, lick, fingerful of food that I put into my mouth. And it helped. A lot. I was amazed at what I was eating that I didn't realize I was eating.

A chart is important because it reveals our patterns with food exactly as they are and not how we imagine them to be. For the next week, and longer if you find it helpful, track your eating habits by keeping a chart.

Exercise 12: Keeping a Chart

As you begin to keep your chart, ask yourself the following questions:

Keeping an eating chart reminds me of _____

_____

When I write down what I eat, I feel as if _____

_____

Eating Chart

Time	Amount	Item	Feelings before eating	Feelings after	Where food was eaten

Eating Chart

Time	Amount	Item	Feelings before eating	Feelings after	Where food was eaten

Eating Chart

Time	Amount	Item	Feelings before eating	Feelings after	Where food was eaten

Eating Chart

Time	Amount	Item	Feelings before eating	Feelings after	Where food was eaten

Chapter 3

Why Weight?

After a lengthy phone conversation with someone who called after reading my first book, *Feeding the Hungry Heart,* I got this note from her: "It's kind of funny to me that in answer to your question 'tell me about yourself,' I could think of nothing more to say beyond, 'I'm a copywriter.' What I really wanted to say was: 'I'm desperate. I'm frightened. I don't want to feel. I hate myself—that's the feeling I know best. I know my problem isn't just fat. At the same time that I've cancelled myself out with food, my life has grown smaller and smaller.' "

When I think about struggling with food, that's the feeling I find most painful: a life that becomes small.

Those of us who are compulsive about food share a common fear: We are afraid that we will never get enough. Of anything. Food. Success. Attention. Love. And one response to that fear is to develop compulsions that protect us from feeling the pain of emptiness: storing and hiding food; eating after we are full; saying "yes" when we want to say "no"; making love when we really don't want to.

We are all interdependent beings; we cannot live or love in total isolation. We need each other. And it's frightening to need, because there is always the chance that we will be starving and no one will answer. When we were children, the fear of emptiness and of being left behind was enough to stop us from opening ourselves. But it's not enough any more. It's not enough because when we close ourselves, cancel ourselves out with food, we are the ones who suffer more than anyone else does. Our lives begin to shrink. And it's not enough because now, as adults, we can

30

choose people who will love us the way we want to be loved (most of the time). When we were children, we didn't have that choice—our families were given to us—but now we can choose the people with whom we can be vulnerable. And it's not enough, because even if we need and no one is there, we will survive.

We are survivors.

We've been abandoned; all of us have molded our personalities around those wounds—bandaged them, protected them from being ripped open again. All of us have known more pain than we thought we could handle. And we handled it. We survived, and we will continue to survive. That is cause for celebration.

Many of us feel that something dark and menacing and unmentionable is wrong with us, and that we have to pay for it forever by binding ourselves to pain, by not allowing ourselves pleasure. Somewhere along the line we missed hearing the message that we were *okay*.

At some point—now—it's a leap of faith. You decide that you're worthy. You decide to let yourself delight in one thing, one sensation that isn't taste. You decide to forget the judgment about your body long enough to remember the brilliance of being alive.

The participants in my workshops ask, "But *how*? How can we allow ourselves pleasure when we feel so unworthy? When we feel fat and ugly and incompetent, when we feel insensitive and selfish—how can we delight in anything, especially our bodies?"

How is becoming aware of the erroneous foundations of your beliefs: how they developed, whose voices they represent, how they are keeping you stuck and at the same time protecting you. *How* is learning what your own voice sounds like—how to say no, how to ask, how to risk. By getting angry. By getting sad. By feeling. *How* is not depriving yourself of foods you love. By eating consciously—when you are hungry, and until you are satisfied.

How is by beginning. Now. I can tell you what I tell the participants in workshops: You are gorgeous. You deserve satisfaction and laughter in your life. You deserve pleasure. You deserve love. I can tell you this a thousand times but you won't believe me until you experience it for yourself. You won't believe me until you begin acting as if you already believe it.

In a Breaking Free workshop last week, someone asked, "When is the little thing going to click that will make it all change?"

Magic. We want magic. We want to be aware for a week or two, to eat when we are hungry for another week or two—and then, it's enough. We want to wake up at our ideal weight, not be troubled by thoughts of chocolate cake, and not ever to binge again. We want those things now. Sooner than now. We want them yesterday.

It's been ten years since I started working on my eating in a conscious, gentle way. Just yesterday I realized that I hadn't written about my body or my weight in my journal for quite a few months. Let's see . . . if I had been waiting for that particular click, I would have waited seven years and seven months after I began eating when I was hungry, six years after I lost thirty pounds, five years after my first book was published, and thirty-seven years and seven months after I was born.

I have a friend, someone I love very much, who has spent the last few years either traveling around the world or in meditation retreats. In four years, she's worked for six months, and those months were spent making enough money to leave. She reminds me of the participants in workshops who keep looking for the answer, keep waiting for the click, and all the while, miss what could be producing it for them: the living of life. Waking up, showering, getting hungry, eating, getting full, talking, working, dreaming, laughing, fighting, loving, crying, sweating, sleeping— and noticing. The boredom, the sadness, the rage, hate, joy, the hunger of being alive. Noticing it all. The ordinary happenings of a day.

This friend of mine keeps opting for the extraordinary in just the way we keep waiting for the magic. We keep thinking something is going to happen that will make it all make sense. And when it doesn't, my friend goes on another retreat or flies to somewhere else in the world. Just as she does, we wait. We wait.

"When is the little thing going to click that will make it all change?"

The answer is that there is no click. Or the answer is that the click is now, here. If you value the experience of getting there instead of the result of being there, one moment is just as good as the next. Learning about your hunger, tasting a raisin as if it were the first you ever ate, stopping when you are satisfied, not stopping and noticing how you feel, it's all part of the process of waking up to being alive.

This book is designed to help you in that process. Allow yourself to be affected by the exercises. Think about them during the days. Talk about them to friends and family.

The important thing is to begin. Now.

There is no reason to wait.

Exercise 13: Hurts from Long Ago

How have you been hurt or abandoned?

EXAMPLES:
1) My mother died when I was three and my dad married a woman who didn't care about my brother or me.
2) My father left after my parents got divorced and I hardly saw him after that.
3) My mom told me that anger was bad, so every time I got angry, I thought *I* was bad.

List the ways in which you've been hurt or abandoned.

1. _____

_____

2. _____

_____

3. _____

_____

4. _____

_____

What did you do to survive that hurt or abandonment?

EXAMPLES:
1) I hid my head under pillows each time I heard my mom and dad screaming at each other.

2) I distracted myself from feeling afraid of my dad's drinking by focusing on the good tastes of food.
3) I made myself hold back the tears each time I felt them in my throat.

List the ways in which you survived being hurt or abandoned.

1. _____

_____

2. _____

_____

3. _____

_____

4. _____

_____

Exercise 14: Do You Believe in Magic?

What are the things that could happen that would change your entire life and make your weight problems disappear forever?

EXAMPLES:
1) I would fall in love, lose weight, and keep it off.
2) By doing the exercises in this book, I will suddenly understand what my problems are about and never struggle again.

Complete the sentence:
The things that could happen that would change my life forever and make me extraordinarily happy are:

1. _____

_____

2. _____

_____

3. _____

_____

4. _____

_____

Exercise 15: If My Weight Could Talk . . .

If your weight could talk, what would it say?

EXAMPLES:
1) It would tell my husband that I am angry with him for telling me to lose weight.
2) It would tell me that I am unhappy with my job and that I want to quit it and start my own business.

Complete the sentence:
If my weight could talk, it would say . . .

1. _____

_____

2. _____

_____

3. _____

_____

4. _____

_____

Exercise 16: My Life Without (This) Weight

What would your life be like if you didn't have a weight problem?

EXAMPLES:
1) My life would be boring. I wouldn't know what to do with my time if I weren't worrying about my body.
2) My life would be perfect. My weight is the only thing that keeps me unhappy.
3) My life would be frightening. I've spent so many years obsessed with food and weight that without it, I have no idea what I could do or think about or talk to my friends about.

Complete the sentence:
Without my conflicts about my body and food, my life would be:

1. _____

_____

2. _____

_____

3. _____

_____

4. _____

_____

Exercise 17: Old Messages

From whom did you get the message that it was unacceptable to be yourself?

Check the appropriate boxes.

_____ mother _____ teacher _____ sister
_____ father _____ grandparent _____ other family member
_____ brother _____ friend _____ lover
_____ religious advisor

List the messages you received.

EXAMPLES:
1) My father told me I was too emotional.
2) My mother told me that I had to keep my mouth shut if I wanted to get married, because men don't like women who think too much.

1. _____

_____

2. _____

_____

3. _____

_____

4. _____

_____

5. _____

_____

6. _____

_____

7. _____

_____

In what ways have you adapted your behavior to conform to those messages?

EXAMPLE:
When my dad told me I was too emotional, I began holding back my feelings and pretending that everything was okay when it really wasn't. I am still pretending.

Complete the sentence:
I've changed myself over the years to conform to the messages I've received about my behavior by:

1. _____

_____

2. _____

_____

3. _____

_____

4. _____

_____

5. _____

_____

6. _____

_____

Exercise 18: Living as If

If you were to decide that you were already absolutely fine the way you are, if you were to begin living as if you deserved love, satisfaction, success, and respect, what would you do? How would you live?

EXAMPLES:
1) I would not feel such a tremendous need to prove myself in everything I did.
2) I would tell people what I think in the moment instead of censoring every thought I have.
3) I would give myself time off every single day to do something I love to do.

Complete the sentence:
If I were to begin living as if I deserved love and satisfaction and all good things, I would:

1. _____

_____

2. _____

_____

3. _____

_____

4. _____

_____

5. _____

_____

• One thing on this list that I will do this week is:

_____

_____

Exercise 19: Beginning Now

Lots of people live as if they were going to live forever, believing that at a certain time in their lives they will finally be ready to give themselves the permission to live the life they've always wanted to live. Lots of people decide that when they get thin, they will finally deserve to live the kind of life they want—and then they spend their lives trying to get thin. And waiting and waiting and waiting to begin living their dreams. Lots of people die without having lived.

This section is designed to help you get in touch with the ways you keep yourself on hold, the dreams you have that you won't let yourself realize because it's not the right time or you're too fat or you don't have the money. This section is designed to help you begin living the life you want. Now.

What are the ways in which you keep yourself from expressing your feelings, from doing what you want to do? What are you waiting for?

Complete the following statements:
If I knew I was going to die next year, I would:

1. _____

_____

2. _____

_____

3. _____

_____

4. _____

_____

• One thing on this list I will do this year is:

_____

_____

If I knew I was going to die next month, I would:

1. _____

_____

2. _____

_____

3. _____

_____

4. _____

_____

• One thing on this list I will do this month is:

_____

_____

If I knew I was going to die tomorrow, I would:

1. _____

_____

2. _____

_____

3. _____

_____

4. _____

_____

• One thing on this list I will do today is:

_____

_____

• Look at your lists and star one thing on each list that you can do in the next three weeks. List each of those things below and specify the week in which you will do it:

1. _____

_____

2. _____

_____

3. _____

_____

CHAPTER 4

Dieting and Bingeing

Diets don't work. They don't work because they treat compulsive eating symptomatically. They assume that the reason people are not thin is because they lack willpower. And that is simply not true. If we lacked willpower, none of us would ever have lost a pound on any diet.

Diets don't work because they assume that we can't trust ourselves, that if we listened to our hunger, we would begin eating at one end of our kitchen and would work our way clear across the United States. Diets don't teach us to listen to the wisdom of our bodies. Diets tell us that our bodies *have* no wisdom, and that if we are to survive, we must control their reckless, bottomless hungers. And that is also untrue.

Diets don't work because they lead to bingeing. For every diet, there is an equal and opposite binge. I have never been on, or heard of, a diet for which there was not a corresponding binge. And that *is* true.

One of my favorite stories about a diet owes its origin to a workshop participant. She and her husband were both on a regulated diet that forbade sweets. On the eighth day of their diet, when she felt that she had-to-have-sugar-and-right-now, she waited for her husband to leave the house, and then assembled the ingredients for an angel food cake. While she was putting the last twirl of icing on the cake, she heard her husband returning. In a panic, she took the cake and shoved it in the clothes dryer. Later that day, he turned on the dryer because his wet socks and shirts were in there. When he bent down, finally, to remove his dry clothes, he found his socks and shirts baked with an angel food cake blown apart in a hundred little pieces.

Diets lead to binges.

Exercise 20: Remembering the Diets

Make a list of all the diets you have been on, beginning with the early ones and finishing with the latest diets you've tried.

Be specific:

    A. What did you eat on those diets?
    B. Did you lose weight?
    C. For how long?
    D. How much weight did you gain when you went off the diet?

EXAMPLE:
I went on a prunes-and-meatball diet for two weeks. I ate nothing but prunes and meatballs; occasionally I ate a hard-boiled egg. I lost seven pounds, but as soon as the diet was over, I binged on ice cream and lasagne and within three days gained eight pounds.

Diet #1:_____

_____

_____

_____

_____

_____

_____

Diet #2: _____

_____

_____

_____

_____

_____

_____

Diet #3: _____

_____

_____

_____

_____

_____

Diet #4: _____

_____

_____

_____

_____

_____

Diet #5: _____

_____

_____

_____

_____

_____

I know that for many of us, five diets will not nearly cover the diets of a lifetime. Over seventeen years, I went on more than thirty diets. Additional space is provided for additional diets.

_____

_____

_____

_____

_____

_____

_____

_____

_____

_____

_____

_____

_____

_____

_____

_____

_____

_____

_____

_____

_____

_____

_____

_____

_____

_____

_____

_____

Look over your list.

Congratulate yourself for the amount of willpower it took to go on all these diets.

Notice the weight you gained by going on diets.

Ask yourself: If diets work, why did I need to go on so many of them?

Exercise 21: Remembering the Binges

Looking back on an eating history that could qualify for the Olympics, I find a few binges to recall with mirth and horror: There was the night my friend Carolyn and I ate two fried chickens, a pound of coleslaw, an entire noodle pudding, and half of a cheesecake. I remember eating a half-gallon of Breyer's vanilla fudge twirl with my fingers in the back of a car when I was twenty-one. And on the day I got a letter from a lover who told me that he no longer wanted to be with me, I went straight to Gayle's bakery and bought—then ate—three cinnamon rolls, two cheese twirls, and three pieces of German chocolate cake. And on and on.

What about you?

On the next page, take time to remember and then list your most memorable binges. Each time you write one down, remember that bingeing is a way of telling yourself that something is wrong and that you need to pay attention to yourself. As you describe the binge, I'd like you also to describe what was going on at the time.

Answer the questions: If the binge could have talked, what would it have said to you? What wasn't working at the time? What did you need that you weren't giving to yourself?

Deprivation

When we feel emotionally deprived, we often try to appease that deprivation by eating. But if what we want is attention, intimacy, solitude, play-time, no amount of food will be enough. It's important for us to examine the ways in which we feel deprived, so that we can ask for what we need and give ourselves what we need directly, in ways that *will be* enough.

The Binge	*What It Might Have Said*
The bakery run after I got the letter from Richard	I was terribly sad and needed to cry. I was also angry, and I needed to express *that*.

The Binge	What It Might Have Said

Exercise 22: What Was I Deprived of?

EXAMPLE:
As a child I felt deprived of consistency and the feeling that I really mattered to anyone in my family.

Complete the sentences:
As a child, I felt deprived of_____

_____

_____

_____

As an adolescent, I felt deprived of_____

_____

_____

_____

_____

As I got older, I felt deprived of_____

_____

_____

_____

_____

_____

_____

Now, I feel deprived of_____

_____

_____

_____

_____

_____

Exercise 23: How I Keep Myself Deprived

As we are growing up, we often have no choices about the ways in which we are deprived. If our parents were distant or unavailable, if we are physically or emotionally abused, we still needed those parents for our survival. We had to stay where we were. But as adults, we have choices. And, too often, we choose to deprive ourselves in the very ways in which we've already *been* deprived.

In the same ways that diets lead to bingeing, because we are depriving ourselves of the foods we like, depriving ourselves on an emotional level also leads to bingeing. When we deprive ourselves of the things we like to do, when we do not allow ourselves pleasure in *daily* (not monthly, not yearly) doses, we turn to food.

How do you keep yourself deprived?

Some examples might be: by not going on vacations; by not taking time for yourself every day; by always being in a rush.

Complete the following list:
I keep myself deprived by:

1. _____

_____

2. _____

_____

3. _____
   _____

4. _____
   _____

5. _____
   _____

6. _____
   _____

7. _____
   _____

Exercise 24: Beliefs about Bingeing

We have many erroneous beliefs about bingeing: that it is brought on by a lack of willpower; that the day after a binge, we must starve ourselves; that once a binge starts, there's no stopping it. There are other ways to treat bingeing: we can regard it as a way of trying to get our own attention. Or we can decide that after a binge, we are going to be kind to ourselves. We can put down our spoons, if only for three seconds, during a binge, and ask ourselves if the food really tastes good—and if we want to go on eating.

Let us examine the erroneous and punitive beliefs we are already holding and discover more tolerant, compassionate counterbeliefs with which we can replace them.

My Beliefs about Bingeing:

EXAMPLES:
1) I believe that when I binge, I lack willpower. A more compassionate belief would be that I am trying to express a feeling that I don't know how to acknowledge directly.

2) I believe that after a binge I should starve myself for a day or two to lose the weight I gained during the binge. A more compassionate belief would be that I take *especially* good care of myself after a binge by eating what I want the next time I get hungry—and stopping when I've had enough.

Complete the sentences:

1. I believe that _____

_____

_____

A more compassionate belief would be that _____

_____

_____

2. I believe that binges are _____

_____

_____

A more compassionate belief would be that _____

_____

_____

3. I believe that the reason I binge is _____

_____

_____

A more compassionate belief would be that _____

_____

_____

4. I believe that after a binge, I should_____

_____

A more compassionate belief would be that_____

_____

5. The next time I binge, I am going to be gentle with myself

and_____

_____

6. On the day after I binge, I am going to be kind to myself

and_____

_____

_____

Exercise 25: Plunges into Oblivion

Binges are ways in which we allow ourselves to go unconscious, to get away from the concerns of day-to-day life and plunge into oblivion for a few minutes. If we developed other ways to meet that need, our desire to binge would lessen.

I believe that we all need to tune out, to retreat or disappear from view at least once a day, and that we ought to make a commitment to ourselves to do this—or else we will become too busy with the shoulds and have-tos to remember the want-tos.

Commit yourself to a fifteen-minute plunge every day. Here are some examples:

Monday: Watch "All My Children."
Tuesday: Read the first two chapters of a novel.
Wednesday: Take an African dance class.

Thursday: See a Katharine Hepburn movie.
Friday: Write in my journal for an hour.
Saturday: Get a facial.
Sunday: Hug and kiss the cat.

It's your turn.

Monday:_____

Tuesday:_____

Wednesday:_____

Thursday:_____

Friday:_____

Saturday:_____

Sunday:_____

Exercise 26: Forbidden Foods

We usually binge on the foods we won't allow ourselves to eat *unless* we binge. It is only when we give ourselves permission to *eat* them that we can choose *not* to eat them. If, for instance, you allow yourself to eat chocolate any time you are hungry for it, then "a chocolate charge" will not build and you won't feel the need to binge on chocolate at a later time. We forbid and forbid and forbid ourselves to have food that we like, food that brings us pleasure. It should be no surprise to us that when we feel a crack in our steely resolve to restrict ourselves—and make a decision to binge—we immediately run for those foods we have not been allowing ourselves to enjoy.

Make a list of the foods you will not allow yourself to eat freely and without guilt. Let yourself think of the food that you determined years ago to shut out of your life, perhaps as far back as childhood. Are sweets included? Bread? Take your time in making the list, remembering foods that you banished, or attempted to banish, or still berate yourself for eating whenever you "succumb":

My Forbidden Foods Are:

_____

_____

_____

_____

_____

_____

_____

_____

_____

Eating My Forbidden Foods

Using the chart on pages 58 and 59, keep a record of what you discover when you do the following:

1. Look at the list you made and decide which is the first food you would like to eat again without guilt.
2. Bring that food into your house this week. Bring more of it than you could possibly eat at one sitting—and *eat it when you are hungry and until you are satisfied*. Allow yourself the pleasure of good tastes.
3. As you eat it, notice whether you like it as much as you thought you would. Notice how it tastes, how it feels in your throat.
4. Remind yourself that you can have it again any time you are hungry.
5. Do the same next week. And the next.
6. Bring one forbidden food into your house each week, until you have no forbidden foods.

Forbidden Foods Chart

Week #	The food I chose from the Forbidden Foods List is:	I bought plenty		I ate it when I was hungry		I stopped when I was satisfied		When I ate it, it, I felt:
		Yes	No	Yes	No	Yes	No	
1								
2								

CHAPTER 5

Eating When You're Hungry

Eating Guideline #1: Eat When You are Hungry.

In any workshop, when I ask participants how they feel about eating when they're hungry, I'll always get one or another or all of these responses:

"If I eat only when I am hungry, I'll never get full enough."

"I can't always *get* food when I am hungry."

"What will I do when I'm through eating?"

"I never let myself get hungry."

"It's not always socially okay to eat where you are when you get hungry."

"If I eat when I'm hungry, it doesn't feel good."

"How do I know when I am hungry?"

"Only skinny people get hungry."

"When I let myself get hungry, I get crabby."

"How can I know the difference between emotional and physical hunger?"

Exercise 27: Feelings about Hunger

What do you think would happen if you ate only when you were physically hungry? Would you eat frequently? Rarely? Would you eat everything in sight (or out of it)?

Complete the following sentence:
If I only ate when I was hungry:

60

EXAMPLES:
1) I would never eat.
2) I would miss eating with friends, at parties, anywhere that was fun.
3) I would get hungry at work and wouldn't be able to eat at my desk.

I would_____

_____

I would_____

_____

I would_____

_____

My friends would_____

_____

My family would_____

_____

Other people would_____

_____

Exercise 28: Eating for the Hunger to Come

Hunger is a survival mechanism. We need to eat to live; our bodies will always let us know when they need food. After years of not listening to the voice of your hunger, I know it's hard for you to believe that you'll get hungry. But you will.

The first step is to wait until you actually get hungry. Most of us don't experience hunger because we don't wait long enough between meals to *get* hungry. We eat for "the hunger to come." We're afraid that if we're going to be somewhere else for three hours, we might get hungry and be stranded some place without anything to eat . . . and then what would happen?

What *would* happen?

If I didn't eat for the hunger to come I might:

1. _____

_____

2. _____

_____

3. _____

_____

Read over the list. Are any of these beliefs true? How do you know?

Exercise 29: Are You Hungry Now? (How Do You know?)

Close your eyes for a minute. Take some long deep breaths in, and let them out. Really let yourself relax. Keep your eyes closed. Roll your tongue around a few times in your mouth. Do you notice any sensations connected with hunger, or fullness, in your mouth? Move your awareness to your throat. Notice those sensations connected with hunger or fullness in your throat. And then, moving your awareness down to your stomach, move one of your hands down to your stomach. No matter what you've eaten or not eaten today, what is your stomach telling you about its need for food? Is *it* hungry? Put your hand on your abdomen (below your navel). Whether you've eaten or not eaten, what is your abdomen telling you? Is *it* hungry?

Exercise 30: What Is Hunger, Anyway?

Circle the part of your body in which you first experience hunger:

throat   abdomen

stomach   head

mouth   legs

Check one of each pair.
Is hunger different from:

pain   _____yes _____no

how?_____

_____

_____

excitement _____yes _____no

how?_____

_____

_____

loneliness _____yes _____no

how?_____

_____

_____

sadness _____yes _____no

how?_____

_____

_____

What feeling follows your recognition that you are hungry?
Circle the answers that apply.

panic   relief   excitement   urgency   fear

Remember that your hunger is your ally. It is your body's
way of telling you that it needs nourishment.

Exercise 31: The Hunger Scale

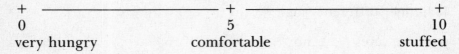

On a scale of 0 to 10, 0 is famished, 10 is "I can't eat another
bite because if I rolled over, my belly would stay on the other
side of the bed." And 5 is comfortable.

With your eyes closed, rate your physical hunger right now. (If
you are at 4 or below, you are hungry; if you are at 5 or above,
you are not.)

At this moment, my hunger is at #____.

For one week, rate your hunger before and after you eat (see
next page). Please do not judge your responses.

Exercise 32: About Meals

For most of our lives, we've eaten at regulated mealtimes called
breakfast, lunch, and dinner. We even have specific times at
which we think these meals should be eaten. However, these
beliefs have little to do with our *bodies'* need for food. Although
it is our bodies that we are feeding, we let our minds decide
what, when, and how much we will eat at any given time.

For the next two days, experiment with your hunger, eating
only in response to your body, and not in response to your
mind's idea of when you should eat. You might eat twice one
day, and seven times the next.

I know that the thought of eating only when you are hungry
might be frightening. Participants in workshops have said things
like: "But what about my family? How will they eat?" and "If I

The Hunger Scale Chart

	Before	*After*
Breakfast		
Lunch		
Dinner		
In-Betweens		
Breakfast		
Lunch		
Dinner		
In-Betweens		
Breakfast		
Lunch		
Dinner		
In-Betweens		
Breakfast		
Lunch		
Dinner		
In-Betweens		
Breakfast		
Lunch		
Dinner		
In-Betweens		
Breakfast		
Lunch		
Dinner		
In-Betweens		
Breakfast		
Lunch		
Dinner		
In-Betweens		

ate ten times a day, people would notice—and would judge me unfairly."

Notice what your reactions are to not eating at meals. And then record them in the space below:

If I don't eat at meals_____

_____

_____

_____

If I don't eat at meals_____

_____

_____

_____

If I eat only when I want to eat_____

_____

_____

_____

Notice how you feel. Hesitation, or fear, of doing something different is natural. But it is not a sign to disregard the exercise. It is only a sign that you are about to do something new and that in so doing, you might precipitate change.

Do you connect certain feelings with mealtimes?
____yes____no
For example, do you associate dinner with being close with your family? ____yes____no
Do you want your hunger to fit into a schedule? ____yes____no

Why?_____

_____

What do you think you would miss if you didn't eat dinner tonight?_____

_____

_____

_____

_____

_____

_____

_____

Exercise 33: The Not-Necessarily-Mealtime Chart

For each day next week, record the times at which you ate and what you ate at those times. How did you feel about eating at that time? What comments did you receive?

A Few Tips:

- If you are not hungry at the time, you can sit at the table with your family while they eat.
- You can bring food with you wherever you go so that you can eat when you are hungry. (Note: If you are not hungry at a specified lunch or dinner break, do something that you'd find pleasurable during that time—and eat later).

Fill in the charts on the following pages.

The Not-Necessarily-Mealtime Chart

Day	Time you ate?	What did you eat?	How did you feel about eating at this time?	What comments did you receive?

The Not-Necessarily-Mealtime Chart

Day	Time you ate?	What did you eat?	How did you feel about eating at this time?	What comments did you receive?

Exercise 34: Eating When You Are Not Hungry

The next few times you eat when you are not hungry, notice:

1. How the food tasted.
2. If you enjoyed it.
3. If it was difficult to know when to stop.
4. If you weren't hungry, what *were* you feeling?

Describe your observations in the space below:

_____

_____

_____

_____

_____

_____

_____

CHAPTER 6

Focusing

Eating Guideline #2: Eat Sitting Down in a Calm Environment
This does not include the car.

Eating Guideline #3: Eat without distractions. Distractions include radio, television, newspapers, books, intense or anxiety-producing conversations, and music.

Although most of us who are compulsive eaters say we love food, my belief is that when you love something you pay attention to it; when you love something, you take time with it. And the way that most of us deal with eating is to distract ourselves from the meal, oblivious to its tastes, its textures, and its smells.

There is a good reason for this: If we're in conflict about the size of our bodies, we believe we don't deserve to eat like "normal" people. We believe that we should be eating cottage cheese and carrot sticks, salad with no dressing, and chicken minus its skin. We believe we have to eat low-calorie foods, if only to prove to ourselves and the world around us that we are, we really are, trying to lose weight. "See?" we tell ourselves. "I may be fat but at least I'm trying. And I deserve credit for that. I deserve credit for *knowing* that I'm unattractive. I may be fat, but I'm not stupid, too."

We don't sit down and enjoy our food because we believe we are not allowed to. We're not allowed to look happy when we eat; we're only allowed to look as if we're trying to lose weight. So what do we do instead? We put on a good show. We eat chicken with the skin removed when "it counts"—when we are

71

sitting down actually eating a meal—and we develop five thousand other ways to eat the foods we really want, while distracting ourselves from the realization that we're eating. We develop ways to eat without really eating, ways to eat that don't count as eating, ways to eat and to lie to ourselves about what we're doing.

We must stop giving ourselves hurtful messages. Now. Not when we lost weight, not when we meet the cultural definition of what is attractive—but NOW. Whether you weigh 105 pounds or 225 pounds, you deserve to have pleasure and joy in whatever you do. Including food. That means oohing and aahing and mmmming about the delights of a meal. That means eating while you sit down in a comfortable and nourishing environment—not in the car or in your bedroom or in the bathroom—and focusing on the wonders of spices and textures and tastes. That means examining all the ways in which you have swallowed falsities about your lack of worth and then standing on a chair and shouting to the whole world: I DESERVE GOODNESS—watch me while I create it.

Let's begin.

Exercise 35: First Reactions

Complete the following sentence:
I can't/don't want to sit down while I eat, and I can't eat without distractions because . . .

EXAMPLES:
1) The only time I get to read is when I eat.
2) If I didn't do anything else while I ate, I would realize how lonely I am when I eat alone.

1. _____

_____

_____

2. _____

_____

_____

3. My family would_____

_____

_____

_____

4. My friends would_____

_____

_____

_____

Exercise 36: Fears

Most of us believe that if we really let ourselves enjoy food, we'd never stop eating. Do you think that?

Complete the sentence:
If I really began enjoying food . . .

1. _____

_____

_____

2. _____

_____

_____

3. _____

_____

_____

4. _____

_____

_____

Eating without Eating

As long as your attention is outside of yourself—on what you are doing, reading, watching—it cannot be inside of you—on the signals that your body is giving you about its hunger and satisfaction levels. When you're reading, you're paying attention to what you are reading about; if you're eating at the same time, the food keeps going in your mouth but you miss the experience of its taste as well as the message that you've had enough. So you're eating without really eating. You're eating without paying attention to, and recognizing, the messages and signals that accompany eating.

The same is true if you pretend that this bite or lick doesn't count. A fine example of this is edging a cake. There have been so many times when I've wanted—and not allowed myself—a piece of cake; what I do instead is notice that the last person who cut herself/himself a piece left ragged edges. It becomes my duty to even them. When I do "edge" it the first time, the cake *still* looks messy, so I have to do it over and over until finally, the two sides—what's left of them—are straight. When I'm finished, I tell myself I haven't had a *piece* of cake: I've only fixed it so that it would look nice. As someone in a workshop said, "It's a hard job, but someone's got to do it."

Exercise 37: Distracted Eating

The ways in which I distract myself from eating are:

1. _____

2. _____

3. _____

4. _____

5. _____

6. _____

7. _____

To add to your own list, here are some of the comments made by workshop participants about their distractions, which include:

- watching television
- reading the newspaper
- cooking
- being on the telephone
- having a difficult discussion
- being in the car

Each time you eat and distract yourself this week, check the distraction—either on your own list or on the one above—that you choose. No judgments. Just awareness.

Exercise 38: Eating That Doesn't Count

Make a list of the ways you eat (i.e., edging a cake) that don't count as eating.

It doesn't count if . . .

1. _____

2. _____

3. _____

4. _____

5. _____

Here are some of the very creative ways in which various workshop participants don't count their eating:

- eating a little chunk of frozen food
- tasting the cake batter before it's baked
- when it's free
- before I exercise
- after I exercise

- if I don't like it
- off the kids' plates
- if no one else sees it
- after sex
- samples at the supermarket

Each time you eat for the next week and don't count it as eating, check the way in which you do it. Again, please don't judge yourself. Just notice what you do.

Exercise 39: Eating in the Car

Car-eating deserves individual mention as a way to eat without really eating. The car used to be my favorite place to eat. It was my dining room, my best kitchen table. I felt safe there. When I would pull up to a stop sign and notice that someone was watching me while I was eating, I'd get furious that they had the nerve to stare. This was my place, and I wanted to be left alone.

If we're trying to distract ourselves from the fact that we're eating, a car is a great place in which to do it because there are so many other things to concentrate on: steering, braking, shifting, stopping, not bumping into the person in front of you, being certain that the person on either side of you knows you are there. And while we're doing all these things, we can quietly demolish a dozen donuts before we stop to realize that we've eaten one. The question is this: Is car-eating the best way to care for yourself, or are you eating in the car because you feel you don't deserve anything better?

Answer these questions:

1. I like eating in my car because_____

_____

_____

_____

_____

2. If I didn't eat in my car, I would miss being able to_____

_____

_____

_____

3. A different way of giving myself what I get from car-eating

might be to_____

_____

_____

_____

4. On _____ [day of the week] of this week, I'll do the above.

Standing at the Refrigerator

A favorite pastime of compulsive eaters. Standing, staring, and eating directly from the refrigerator. I don't call it eating; I call it grazing.

Exercise 40: The Two of You

Imagine inviting a friend for dinner. When she arrives, tell her that she'll be joining you at your favorite table—the refrigerator. And that you will be standing, not sitting, for dinner.

Complete the sentences:

1. I think my guest would_____

_____

_____

_____

2. As her hostess, I would feel_____

_____

_____

3. When I think of standing and eating at the refrigerator in this

light, I_____

_____

When we stand at the refrigerator to eat, we make a statement to ourselves that we are not our own best guests. Is that a statement you want to make?

The next time you find yourself standing and eating at the refrigerator—pull up a chair. That way, you'll give yourself the message that you are really eating. If someone walks in the door and asks you what you are up to, tell them sweetly and simply that you're eating!

Exercise 41: Real Eating

If standing at the refrigerator isn't real eating and eating in the car isn't real eating, if edging a cake isn't real eating—then what is?

Complete the sentences:

1. Real eating is_____

_____

_____

2. On _____ [day of the week] of this week, I am going to treat myself well and eat in a way that I consider "real eating."

The way I am going to do that is_____

_____

Exercise 42: Be Your Own Guest

1. Choose one time this week when you can eat by yourself.
2. Set the table with your best silverware, glassware, or dishes. Use cloth napkins and candles.
3. Serve yourself food that you really like. Make this a special meal, a meal that you would serve to a loved one.
4. Before you eat, notice the aroma of the food; try to distinguish between one spice and the next. Look at the food. Notice its color.
5. Take one bite and eat it slowly. Very slowly. How does the taste change as you chew? How does the food feel against the roof of your mouth? On your tongue?
6. Eat the next bite exactly as you ate the first one, noticing the exquisite combinations of taste, color and texture.
7. Eat the meal, enjoying it to the fullest in whatever way feels most pleasurable and comfortable to you.
8. When you're finished with the meal, answer these questions:
   a. When I used my best table setting for myself, I felt:
   ____uncomfortable ____comfortable ____very glad

   other_____
   b. When I sat down to this meal, I:
   ____wanted it to be over with.
   ____looked forward to eating every bite.

   other_____
   c. When I ate slowly, the food tasted:
   ____terrible ____okay ____delicious
   d. After the meal, I:
   ____wanted more food ____felt satisfied ____was thrilled

   e. By eating this way, I learned that_____

   _____

   _____

CHAPTER 7

Eating What You Want

Eating Guideline #4: Eat Only What You Want.

Those of us who know only how to diet or binge translate
"eat-what-you-want" into "permission-to-binge." This guideline
is heard as: "Eat what you want whenever you want it and as
much of it as you can possibly eat in one sitting."
    What do you hear?"

Exercise 43: Immediate Reactions

What do you feel when you hear that you can eat what you want?

Circle one response:

scared   panicked   glad   ecstatic   relieved   suspicious

And complete the following sentences:

I feel _____ when I hear that I can eat what I want

because_____

_____

If I eat what I want, I will_____

_____

_____

Exercise 44: Foods I (Think I) Want

We often want things, people, situations that we think we can't have. This holds true for food. When you imagine yourself eating what you want, what kinds of foods are in your mind's eye?

These are the foods I want:

1. _____

2. _____

3. _____

4. _____

5. _____

6. _____

7. _____

8. _____

9. _____

Exercise 45: The Seduction of Wanting

When I was about six, a major toy company produced a doll called Patti Playpal. Patti was three feet high, had bright blue eyes, and cost twenty-six dollars. I wanted her. My mother said, "That's too expensive. Absolutely no." I was crushed. I dreamed about her for months, convinced that if only I could have a Patti Playpal, my life would be perfect. On my birthday, Patti was waiting for me at the kitchen table. She was dressed in a blue-and-white checked pinafore, white lace socks, and black patent leather shoes. I was thrilled. For two days. And then I left her in a corner of my room, bright-eyed and lonely, to keep company with the stuffed poodle.

Consider the things you have wanted—and received—in your life. What did you believe would happen when you got them? And then, what actually *did* happen?

Things I have wanted and received:
As a child:

1. _____

2. _____

3. _____

4. _____

5. _____

As a teenager:

1. _____

2. _____

3. _____

4. _____

5. _____

As an adult:

1. _____

2. _____

3. _____

4. _____

5. _____

Exercise 45: The Reality of Having

Pick one of your responses from childhood, one from your teenage years, and one from your adult life and describe how having what you wanted changed your feelings about it:

1. As a child, I thought that having_____

_____would_____

_____.

I discovered instead that_____

_____

_____.

2. As a teenager, I thought that having_____

_____would_____

_____

_____.

I discovered instead that_____

_____

_____.

3. As an adult, I thought that having_____

_____would_____

_____.

I discovered instead that_____

_____

_____.

Exercise 47: Food *Is* Only Food

When we realize that we can have the foods we want, the need and desire to have them *all the time* disappear. If we can have them whenever we're hungry for them, they lose their power and become ordinary.

Buy one food that you want and have not allowed yourself to eat.

After you finish eating it, answer the following questions:
1. Once I bought the food and ate it without guilt, did I still want it as much as I thought I had?

_____yes   _____no

2. If I felt that I could eat this food as much as I wanted it—as much, say, as I feel I can eat carrots or lettuce—would my desire for this food change?

_____yes   _____no

We can only give ourselves permission *not* to eat when we give ourselves permission *to* eat. We can only tell the difference between foods that we want and foods that we think we want when we give ourselves permission to eat *all* foods.

Exercise 48: What Do I Really Want?

The first step in eating what you want is deciding what you truly want.

To decide what you want to eat:

1. You must first be hungry. If you aren't, then it will be your mind that is making decisions, not your body. And since it's your body that you're feeding, it's important to listen to the cues it gives you.
2. Sit down for thirty seconds or a minute.
   a. See if you get an image of a particular food—i.e., an egg salad sandwich, a piece of pizza.

     b. Notice if you can taste or smell a particular food (without, of course, having it in front of you).
     c. If the answer to either of these questions is yes, that is the food your body is wanting at the moment.
3. If you still don't know what food you want, ask yourself these questions:

Do I want something . . .
- spicy
- sweet
- bland

Do I want something . . .
- hot
- cold
- at room temperature

Do I want something . . .
- crunchy
- smooth

For the coming week, fill out the chart on pages 86, every time you get hungry.

Calories Don't Count

They don't.

And I'll tell you why: When you eat what you want to eat, you can stop eating when you've had enough. When you eat by counting calories, you figure that you've been so good—after all, celery *burns* calories—why not eat a little more? And a little more. Soon you've consumed more calories than you might have if you'd begun with exactly what you wanted in the first place.

Remember that it is only when you give yourself permission to eat that you can give yourself permission not to eat. When you give yourself permission to eat the foods you love, you can give yourself permission not to eat them when you're hungry for something else (i.e., emotional release, time alone, affection).

What Do I Want to Eat?

Am I Hungry?		Do I get a picture of or a feeling for what I want to eat?		Do I smell or taste what I want to eat?		Do I want something . . . (check one or more)									What then will I eat?
YES	NO	YES	NO	YES	NO	spicy	sweet	bland	cold	hot	room temp.	smooth	crunchy	other	

What Do I Want to Eat?

Am I Hungry?		Do I get a picture of or a feeling for what I want to eat?		Do I smell or taste what I want to eat?	Do I want something... (check one or more)									What then will I eat?
NO	YES	NO	YES	NO	YES	spicy	sweet	bland	cold	hot	room temp.	smooth	crunchy	other	

Restaurant Eating, Social Eating

When you go to a restaurant and are presented with a varied menu, it's still important to check with your body and see what *it* wants. Ask yourself the questions about taste, temperature, and texture—then choose.

If you go to a friend's house and she/he has cooked dinner and you don't like anything being served, you can:

1. Tell the truth.
2. Swirl your food around on your plate and make it look as though you are eating it.
3. Eat a little of it; then when you get home, you can eat what you really want.

On Leftovers, Doggie Bags, etc.

There have been many times at restaurants when I've eaten exactly what and how much I wanted to eat and then taken the rest home. I am very disappointed when the next day I discover that my body does not want what is in the bag.

Part of eating what you want to eat is recognizing that your tastes change from meal to meal and certainly from day to day.

Be willing to be surprised.

And enjoy yourself.

CHAPTER 8

About Satisfaction

Eating Guideline #5: Eat Until You Are Satisfied.

Satisfaction is different from fullness. Satisfaction is: "I can stop eating now. I may still have room for more food but I'm at a comfortable stopping place." Fullness is: "I can't eat another bite." True hunger is physical; satisfaction is both emotional and physical. Being hungry depends on what you last put into your body and when you did so. Being satisfied depends not only on when and what (and how much) you eat, but on your *feelings* about what you eat.

There are certain prerequisites for being satisfied:

1. You must be hungry when you begin eating. If there was no signal to begin, there will be no signal to end.
2. You must eat what you want to eat. If you are eating foods that you don't want, either because they are low in calories or because they are free or leftover or you paid for them, etc., you will not be emotionally satisfied. You won't feel good about either yourself or the meal and you will leave wanting more. You may be physically full, but you will still want more.
3. Your attention must be present. Satisfaction is a result of being in the present moment. If you are reading or watching television, if you are distracting yourself in some way from the taste of the food and from how it feels in your body, you will completely miss the signal of satisfac-

89

tion that your body gives you. That signal is soft, unlike hunger and unlike fullness, and you must be listening to hear it.

4. To stop eating when you are satisfied and before you are uncomfortably full, you must believe that you can eat again when you're hungry. If you think this is your last chance to eat a particular food or your last chance to eat what you want, you will try to store good tastes by eating more than enough. If you threaten yourself by promising yourself that you will diet on Monday, or on New Year's Day, or three weeks before your sister's wedding, or if Breaking Free doesn't work, you will eat to defend against the deprivation to follow.

5. Stopping when you are satisfied may mean not finishing the food on your plate. It means being willing to "waste food"; it means being willing to put food away, throw it away, or give it away. It means resigning from the clean-plate club.

Exercise 49: The Hunger Scale and Satisfaction

On the hunger scale (see Chapter 5, page 64), satisfaction is the number at which you feel comfortable stopping. Remember that satisfaction is relative. What is satisfying to you one day might not be enough to satisfy you the next.

When I first began following the Eating Guidelines, I was unsure of being able to figure out what I wanted to eat and then to stop when I had enough. I couldn't remember *any* time that I had had *enough* food. So I experimented with satisfaction levels.

For the first few months, I didn't trust myself to eat whenever I got hungry; I was positive that at any moment, I would put myself back on a diet, and so I consistently ate more than my body needed to protect myself against future deprivation. Satisfaction, therefore, was a feeling of fullness. On the hunger scale, it was number 7; sometimes I didn't feel satisfied until my level of fullness had reached number 8.

As I began to listen to my body's needs, I felt comfortable with eating less, knowing that if I got hungry an hour later, I would allow myself to eat whatever I wanted. I was then able to stop eating at number 5 on the scale. Number 5 is the point at which you feel yourself getting full, but are not full *yet*.

After I had learned to call a halt at number 5, I was ready to feel a little lighter when I stopped eating. I wanted to feel as if I could get up and dance after I ate, so I practiced stopping at number 3 and number 4 on the scale. Number 3 was uncomfortable; I was still a little hungry. Number 4 felt just right. I was no longer hungry; my body seemed light and I was satisfied with what I had eaten. Most of the time now, I stop eating at number 4, though there are times when being there doesn't feel like I've had enough food. Depending on the season, or on how I am feeling physically and emotionally, my need for the type and quantity of food changes—and I eat accordingly.

What amount of food feels satisfying to you *today*?

1. Next time you eat, rate yourself on the hunger scale. And complete the following sentence:

   I was satisfied today when I stopped eating at number___.

   I knew I was satisfied because_____

   _____

   _____

   _____

2. After you eat a meal on Tuesday of next week, rate yourself on the hunger scale. And complete the following sentence:

   I was satisfied today at number ___ when I stopped eating.

   I knew I was satisfied because_____

   _____

   _____

   _____

3. After you eat a meal one month from today, rate yourself on the hunger scale. And complete the following sentence:

I was satisfied and stopped eating today at number ___. I

knew I was satisfied because_____

_____

_____

_____

Practice Exercises

If you have been on diets or eating compulsively for very long, you probably feel that you *can't* get satisfied. (Remember that the message of diets is that your hunger is bottomless and that if you let yourself eat what you want without strict rules, you would devour everything in sight.)

Here are some exercises to help you get acquainted with satisfaction:

1. Eat half the food on your plate and then check to see where you are on the hunger scale.

   Complete the following sentence:
   After eating half the food on my plate, I am at number ___ on the hunger scale.

2. If you are at number 5 or above, stop eating.

   Complete the following sentence:
   When half the food on my plate is left and I stop eating,

   I_____

   _____

3. Make a list of all the beliefs you have about throwing food away or wasting food.

EXAMPLES:
a. I have to eat all the food on my plate because children are starving in India/Africa/South America.
b. Throwing food away is wasteful.

My beliefs about not finishing the food on my plate are:

1. _____

_____

2. _____

_____

3. _____

_____

4. _____

_____

Helpful Hints about Waste:

• A woman in a workshop said: "You either throw it out or you throw it in."
• If you have had enough food and continue to eat, it turns to waste either inside your body or outside it.
• If you are in the middle of a meal and you don't know whether you are satisfied or not you can:
  a. push your plate away
  b. go to another room
  c. do anything that breaks the hand-to-mouth momentum and gives you the opportunity to check in with your body
• Notice the difference between fullness and satisfaction; pay close attention to how each of them feels and begin to practice whichever feels better. Remember that there is no right or

wrong. If you are more comfortable always being full and if you find that being full is synonymous with being satisfied, that is absolutely fine.

Complete the following sentences:

When I'm full, I feel_____

_____

I like being full because_____

_____

I don't like being full because_____

_____

Being satisfied is/isn't different from being full because_____

_____

I like being satisfied because_____

_____

I don't like the feeling of satisfaction because_____

_____

CHAPTER 9

About Sneaking

Eating Guideline #6: Eat (with the Intention of Being) in Full View of Others.

Someone I once worked with told this story: "I love potato chips, but I feel I shouldn't eat them. I'm too fat and potato chips have so many calories; if anyone saw me eating them, they'd be disgusted. So I have devised a method of eating them without being seen: I take the bag and a pair of scissors into my bedroom. I close the door and get under the covers and pile even more blankets on top of me. Then I snip the top of the bag, take one out and suck on it—I can't crunch because what if someone in the house hears me? This way, I get to eat potato chips and no one ever knows."

Exercise 50: Ways I Sneak

"Eating with the intention of being in full view" means not sneaking. If you eat alone, it means not being afraid that someone will walk in the door and see what you're eating. It means telling the truth about the food you eat.

How do you sneak food?

EXAMPLES:
1) By eating modest amounts of food at a party, then coming home and eating a meal.
2) By running back and forth to the kitchen (and eating) while people are in the living room.

95

3) By ordering a cake at the bakery for yourself and telling the cashier that it is for your kids.

Complete the sentence:
I sneak food by:

1. _____

_____

_____

2. _____

_____

_____

3. _____

_____

_____

4. _____

_____

_____

5. _____

_____

_____

Exercise 51: Why I Sneak

Why do you sneak?

EXAMPLES:
1) I sneak because if people saw what I ate, they'd think I was a pig.

2) If I didn't, I'd never get to eat what I want.

Complete the sentences:
I sneak because . . .

1. _____

_____

_____

_____

2. If I didn't_____

_____

_____

_____

3. It helps me to_____

_____

_____

_____

4. Without it, I would_____

_____

_____

_____

5. It protects me from_____

_____

_____

_____

The Message of Sneaking

Whenever you tell yourself something about your body, you hear it on an emotional level as well. For instance, when you tell yourself that you have to diet because otherwise you'd eat everything in sight, the message you hear is that your hungers are bottomless—all your hungers, including your hunger for intimacy, for self-expression, for play, or for solitude. You cannot separate the physical part of you from the emotional part of you.

The message you give yourself when you sneak is: "If the people in my life saw me, they wouldn't love me. Who I am is unlovable, too needy. I cannot reveal myself. If I want to be loved, I must hide."

Exercise 52: If They Really Knew

Is there someone special in your life that you feel would be disappointed if she/he knew what and how much you ate?

Complete the following sentences:

1. If _____ [name of person] knew what I ate, he/she would_____

_____

_____

_____

2. If _____ [name] knew what I ate, he/she would_____

_____

_____

_____

_____

3. If _____ [name of person or group of people] knew

what I ate, they would_____

_____

_____

_____

Exercise 53: Judgments

Lots of people are afraid that if they let others see what they eat, they'd get reactions like, "But what about that diet?" or "Didn't you say you wanted to lose weight? How can you be eating creme puffs?"

It's important for you to remember that most people who struggle with food and their weight believe that they must diet to lose weight. When they see you eating exactly what you want, they are likely to feel confused, angry, envious, self-righteous. After all, if it's possible to reach a desirable weight without dieting, why are they suffering so on their diets? Judgments have much more to do with the person who is making them than the person to whom they refer.

A corollary of this is that we often feel that people are judging us when in truth we are judging ourselves. If we feel uncomfortable or ashamed of eating in front of other people, we'll place that discomfort outside ourselves and believe that someone else thinks we're doing something wrong.

What are the horrible things you say to yourself when you eat exactly what you want to eat?

1. _____

_____

_____

_____

2. _____

_____

_____

3. _____

_____

_____

_____

What are the worst things people could say if they saw you eating what you want to eat?

Complete the sentences:
The worst possible things are:
1. _____

_____

_____

2. _____

_____

_____

3. _____

_____

_____

_____

Now, think about replies you could make.

EXAMPLES:
1. "I know you think I shouldn't be eating this, but I'm on a new program. I'd like your support."
2. "You think this is a lot? You should have seen what I ate for lunch!"
3. "How do *you* feel about eating what you want? I suspect that your judgments about me have to do with your judgments about yourself. Would you like to talk about it?"

Complete the sentences:

If someone told me that_____

_____, I would

reply that_____

_____

If someone told me that_____

_____

I would reply that_____

_____

Practice these replies prior to any occasion on which you are likely to be judged: before going out with friends, before parties, before family gatherings.

Exercise 54: Making the Commitment

When I first started to eat what I wanted, I made a commitment to myself that I would not sneak food. This was a difficult commitment to make—and keep—because most of the eating I *did* was sneak-eating. I was ashamed of myself; I was ashamed of what I looked like, what I ate, what I felt. Sneaking, I knew from experience, was humiliating. But I knew that the only way to begin feeling better about myself was to practice treating myself with dignity and respect.

To stop sneaking, you must make a commitment to yourself that you will stop—and then keep that commitment. Two times this week, decide that you will not sneak at a time when you would ordinarily have done so. And then answer the following questions:

1. Was *not* sneaking harder than I thought it would be?

    ____yes   ____no

2. During the experience, I felt:

    ____uncomfortable   ____proud of myself   ____indifferent

3. Next week, I can make a commitment not to sneak __(#) times.

Thoughts on Commitment

I find it helpful to distinguish between commitment and discipline.

The message I give myself when I feel that I ought to be disciplined is that I am unorganized, lazy, and wild. Because that message isn't a kind one, I react against it. I dislike being told (even by myself) that I can't be regulated, that I can't be trusted to accomplish what is important to me. I rebel—and do exactly what I've told myself I must *not* do.

The message I give myself when I make a commitment to something or someone is that I am aware of wanting to act in a certain way or reach a particular goal; I am in touch with my power and ability to act on that power. The feeling-tone of the word commitment is one of self-respect; it communicates the belief that my actions will reflect my values and desires and that I believe in myself.

Discipline and diets lead to binges.

Commitment and self-trust lead to change.

CHAPTER 10

On Being Joyful, With Food and Without

Eating Guideline #7: Eat with Enjoyment, Gusto, and Pleasure.

Last summer, I brought fresh-picked blackberries to my two-and-a-half-year-old friend Sasha's house. We made sourdough blackberry pancakes together and then sat down to eat them. Within two minutes, Sasha's face looked like a blackberry. She had blackberry eyebrows, blackberry eyelashes, blackberry cheeks. She was squealing with delight, rubbing the pancake in her hair, and pounding it on her rubber placemat with glee. She was having fun.

We adults, on the other hand, take eating so s-e-r-i-o-u-s-l-y. We are concerned with our manners, with not being messy, with not dripping or spilling foods, with not leaving traces of salad in our teeth.

Remember when you took the insides out of white bread and rolled them into a thick pasty ball? When you opened your mouth as you were eating peanut butter and showed your brother/sister/friend how it stuck to your tongue? Remember when you let the ice cream melt and swirled it around and around in your bowl? Remember when you used to have FUN with food?

Exercise 55: Playing with Food

I'm not suggesting that you rub blackberries on your eyebrows or throw pizza at the wall. I am suggesting that you see the food on your plate as an opportunity to let the child-part of you come out.

If I decided to have fun with my food, I would:

EXAMPLES:
1) make a cake in the shape of the Empire State Building.
2) create an all-white meal.
3) use food coloring to make orange broccoli and purple mashed potatoes.

Complete the sentence:
If I decided to have fun with my food, I would:

1. _____

_____

_____

2. _____

_____

_____

3. _____

_____

_____

4. _____

_____

_____

5. On _____ [day of the week] of this week, I will play with

my food by_____

_____

_____.

Suggestions:

- One day this week, pick a meal and eat blindfolded. Notice the taste, texture. What is it like to eat food and not be able to see it? What senses become dominant?
- To be done with someone you love and trust: Eat a meal during which you are silent and can only eat by pointing to what you want and allowing yourself to be fed.
- Eat a meal with your fingers—no silverware at all. Notice how your appreciation of the food changes when you touch it. Do you like it? Do you feel like a kid again?

Exercise 56: Your Childlike Self

Sometimes in a workshop, I'll say, "Who here likes to be *bad*?" And suddenly I see gleaming eyes, mouths turned up at the corners. I hear snickers and giggles and guffaws. Everyone likes to let the child inside come out, but he won't do it often enough.

Take a moment and consider the qualities in you that are joyful and childlike.

Complete the sentence:
The child in me is:
EXAMPLE: mischievous and talks in a funny voice.

1. _____

2. _____

3. _____

4. _____

Exercise 57: Noticing the Lost Parts

What joyful parts of yourself have you given up as you've gotten older?

EXAMPLES:
1) singing as much as I'd like
2) making spontaneous decisions—and acting on them

Complete the sentence:
As I've gotten older, I've given up:

1. _____

2. _____

3. _____

4. _____

Exercise 58: Reclaiming the Lost Parts

How might you let the child inside you express herself/himself?

EXAMPLES:
1) I could stomp in rain puddles.
2) I could take a bubble bath in the middle of the day.

Complete the sentences:
If I let myself be childlike, I would:

1. _____

2. _____

3. _____

4. _____

This week, decide that you will do three joyful, childlike activities that you wouldn't ordinarily do. After you do each one, complete the following statements:

My first activity was_____

After I did it, I felt_____

_____

The second way in which I created joy for myself this week

was_____

_____

As I was doing it, I felt_____

_____

The third way I let the child in me come out was_____

_____

I learned that_____

_____

More Suggestions:

- Throw a surprise party for someone whose birthday it isn't.
- Go on a picnic, red-checked table cloth and everything, in the middle of the living room.
- Write a personal ad to someone you love for a paper she/he reads.
- Do something you've always wanted to do. Take horseback riding lessons. Learn to play the harmonica.
- Let go of your routine for a week. Eat breakfast at dinner time.
- Tell the maître d' that it's your friend's birthday when it isn't. Watch her face when twenty-six waiters serenade her.

Exercise 59: If I Had It to Do Over

A few years ago I read a piece by Nadine Stair called "If I Had It to Do Over," in which she was looking back on her life as an older woman and remarking about the things she would do differently. Some of the things she said were: "I would wear more purple; I would eat fewer beans and more ice cream; I would go barefoot earlier in spring."

　　And you? If you were eighty-five years old right now and you were looking back on the life you had lived, what would you want to do differently?

EXAMPLES:
1) I would want to take money less seriously.
2) I would want to tell the people I love that I love them.
3) I would want to take more vacations.

Complete the sentences:
If I had it to do over, I would:

1. _____

_____

2. _____

_____

3. _____

_____

4. _____

_____

5. _____

_____

6. _____

_____

7. _____

_____

Of the seven items you listed, which ones can you begin doing this month?

Complete the sentence:
This month, I will:

1. _____

_____

2. _____

_____

3. _____

_____

Exercise 60: One Birthday Is Not Enough

My birthday always came at the end of the summer after camp and before school.

No one ever knew it was my birthday (except my parents, of course, for whom the day had a certain ring), and consequently, I didn't get the attention I thought any self-respecting kid should get. Not to mention the presents.

So, in my first year of college, my friend Jace and I conspired to give ourselves new birthdays and throw each other parties to celebrate them. It worked. Every year for four years, I celebrated my birthday in August and then again in November.

I'm thinking of reinstituting that system. One birthday is simply not enough.

Answer the following questions:
If today were your birthday . . .
1. What would you do?

_____

_____

_____

2. With whom would you celebrate?

_____

3. What would ask for?

_____

_____

4. What would you give yourself?

_____

_____

Why not live as if today is your birthday?
Why not live as if every day is your birthday?
Why not?

CHAPTER 11

Working with Pain

Pain hurts. No one likes to be in pain. No matter what we try to do to avoid it, however, sometimes we can't help but give or get hurt. People we love get sick; someone we love doesn't love us; things don't turn out the way we planned; people we love die.

There is pain. And there is our reaction to it.

Compulsive eating is a reaction to pain. If we are to stop eating compulsively, we must discover new ways to deal with, express, or avoid our pain.

When you are in pain, you are probably feeling one or a combination of the following:

hurt	guilt	grief
fear	confusion	shame
anger	jealousy	worry
sadness	loneliness	rejection

Exercise 61: The Color of Pain

When we were very small, the world seemed very big. Feelings seemed gigantic. Pain felt as though it would rip us apart if we let ourselves really experience its depth. So we didn't. We shut it off. We ate.

Few of us have ever taken the time to examine what pain is, what it feels like, where it is located in our bodies, whether it is bigger than we are. Our first reaction to pain is to avoid it. We are still operating from the child-belief that we are very small and pain is so big that we must not let ourselves feel it.

In the space below, draw a picture of your pain. Use crayons. Then answer the following:

What color is your pain?
What shape is your pain?
Is it bigger or smaller than you?

What else do you observe when you look at your drawing?
Comments:

_____

_____

_____

_____

_____

_____

Exercise 62: Old Pain, Past Pain

As children, we ate to take care of ourselves, protect ourselves, deal with our pain in a way that was quick, easy, and self-sufficient.
   What were some of the pains you ate to avoid or express when you were a child?

Complete the following sentences:
When I was a child, I was in pain about:

EXAMPLES:
1) being sent to my aunt's house when my mother died when I was ten. Everyone told me my mom was in heaven and that I should be glad she was an angel but no one told me it was okay to be sad.
2) my father calling me selfish when I asked for a second bathing suit after wearing my old one for two years.

1. I was in pain* about_____

_____

_____

*This may include times when you felt ashamed, frustrated, confused, uncomfortable, or upset.

2. _____

_____

_____

3. _____

_____

_____

4. _____

_____

_____

Exercise 63: Fears about Pain

What do you think would happen if you let yourself *feel* your pain—instead of eating it away?

Some people say:

"I'd never stop crying."
"It would take me over."
"I'd want to stay in bed all day."

Complete the following sentence:
If I let myself experience my pain, I would:

1. _____

_____

_____

2. _____

_____

_____

3. _____

_____

_____

4. _____

_____

_____

Exercise 64: Present Pain

What in your life are you in pain about now?

Complete the sentence:
In my life right now, I'm in pain about:

1. _____

_____

_____

2. _____

_____

_____

3. _____

_____

_____

4. _____

_____

_____

Exercise 65: What to Do with Pain

Examine a recent time in the past when you ate as a reaction to being in pain.

Complete the following sentences:

I ate when I was in pain as a reaction to:_____

_____

_____

I ate because I felt that if I *didn't* eat, I would_____

_____

_____

As a result of eating: (check one)
—The pain went away forever.
—The pain got worse.
—I forgot what I was in pain about.
—I felt much better about myself.
—I felt terrible about myself.
—The pain came back the next day.

At best, eating can numb us, soothe us, distract us from the source of our pain. There *are* more direct and satisfying ways to express our pain, ways that reaffirm our strength and ability to handle the crises that life is always dishing out.

Here are alternative ways of dealing with pain. Check the ones that you could do:

—cry   —read an inspirational book
—take a walk   —draw a picture of my pain
—call a friend   —lie down with a heating pad
—hit a pillow   —take a bubble bath
—write in my journal   —ask to be held
—listen to soothing music —sit in a rocking chair

Exercise 66: Making Changes

After checking the different ways of handling your pain, make a commitment to yourself to go through with one of them.

Complete the sentences:

The last time I was in pain, I_____

_____

_____

_____

The next time I am in pain, I will_____

_____

_____

_____

Another time I am in pain, I will_____

_____

_____

_____

When I am in pain again, I will_____

_____

_____

_____

Allowing Misery

When we are miserable, it is important to let ourselves be miserable. In a book called *I Like You* by Sandol Stoddard Warburg (Boston: Houghton Mifflin, 1965), the author says, "I like you because/When I am feeling sad/You don't always cheer me up right away/Sometimes it is better to be sad/ . . . You want to think about things/It takes time."

Let yourself be sad, miserable, unhappy, in pain.

Decide that for a limited amount of time every day, say fifteen minutes, you are going to do nothing but feel miserable.

Can you spend fifteen whole minutes being nothing but miserable? Try it.

Then complete the following:

After setting aside fifteen minutes to be miserable, I:

EXAMPLES:
1) discovered that fifteen minutes was a long time.
2) finally let myself cry about how lonely I've felt this week.

1. _____

_____

2. _____

_____

3. _____

_____

CHAPTER 12

Judgments and Anger

A few years ago I went on a meditation retreat at which the teacher asked us to be aware of the judgments we made in a period of three hours. At the end of that time, I laughed (to myself, of course, for this was a silent retreat); I realized that I had judgments about everything: smiles, teeth, legs, socks, hair. Even without eye contact (for this was an eyes-down retreat) and conversation, I had decided which people I liked and which people I didn't like.

It was amusing to catch myself in the act of judging. But there is something terribly serious about judging other people: It is an unequivocal sign that we judge ourselves. And harshly.

We judge ourselves because *we've been judged*—by people important to us, by people we thought knew better than we did, by people whose opinions we trusted. We judge ourselves because we believe that if we didn't, we would let ourselves off scot-free and never change. We judge ourselves because we are afraid of what would happen and who we would become if we didn't.

Judgments serve no purpose except to keep us feeling inadequate. They do not lead to change. They do not lead to openness. They do not lead to love. They do not lead to thinness. If they did, every single one of us would be thin by now.

Remember that *whenever* you are judging someone else, no matter what the circumstances are, the person you are truly judging is yourself. No matter what.

Exercise 67: Judging Yourself

What do you judge (negatively) about yourself?

Make a list:

1. _____

_____

2. _____

_____

3. _____

_____

4. _____

_____

5. _____

_____

6. _____

_____

7. _____

_____

Exercise 68: My Most Unforgivable Thoughts/Actions

What is so terrible about you that you feel in constant need of judgment? What have you thought, felt, done, that is unforgivable?

EXAMPLES:
1) I thought about killing my brother when he was younger.
2) I lied to my husband when I told him I was not having an affair.

Complete the sentence:
My most unforgivable thought/action-feelings are:

1. _____

_____

2. _____

_____

3. _____

_____

4. _____

_____

Read each one of them aloud. After each one, say, "I forgive you" to yourself. Do this once a day for a week or as long as it feels healing.

Exercise 69: A Life Without Judgments

What would happen, what would you do, how would you act if you stopped judging yourself today?

EXAMPLE:
I would stop trying to guess what someone's reaction will be to what I say—and I might begin telling the truth.

1. _____

_____

_____

2. _____

_____

_____

3. _____

_____

_____

4. _____

_____

_____

How did you feel as you wrote the above list?
Did you feel happy? Frightened? Relieved?
Star one thing on that list that you could do NOW.

Exercise 70: When Do You Get Judgmental?

During what times or in what situations do you begin judging
yourself?

EXAMPLE:
Whenever I enter a roomful of people, I begin feeling as though I
have nothing important to say, so I stay by myself and feel left out.

Complete the sentence:
I begin judging myself when:

1. _____

_____

2. _____

_____

3. _____

_____

4. _____

_____

Exercise 71: Instead of Judging

What could you do instead of judging yourself at these times?
What kinds of things could you say to yourself?

EXAMPLE:
I could make a promise to myself to talk to two people when I
get into a group. And I could keep the promise.

Complete the sentence:
Instead of judging myself, I could:

1. _____

_____

_____

2. _____

_____

_____

3. _____

_____

_____

4. _____

_____

_____

NOTE: When you notice that you are judging yourself, acknowledge what you are doing and let it go. Don't judge your judging.

About Anger

Most of us are frightened of our anger. We received messages a long time ago that anger was bad, or that if we expressed our anger we would be punished or hurt someone. There is nothing wrong with anger. It's a natural response to a situation in which you feel violated in some way. Getting angry is a way of saying, "You've reached my limits. Don't push any further," or "You've hurt me and I'm afraid that you don't care about me."

We become frightened of our anger when we do not honor it. We become frightened of our anger when we swallow it and pretend everything is fine when it isn't.

In the moment, however, anger is simply anger. It flames inside us, and if we express it, it passes. If we are very angry, it may take longer for the feelings to pass, but they will. All feelings do.

Exercise 72: Anger "Leftovers"

Anger seethes inside us when we do not express it. It doesn't go away by itself. It is important that we acknowledge our anger leftovers so that when we get angry in the present, our anger is not also fed by the years we didn't allow ourselves to express it.

Who in your past are you angry with? And for what?

Complete the sentences:

1. I am angry with_____for_____

_____

_____

2. I am angry with_____for_____

_____

_____

3. I am angry with_____for____

_____

_____

4. I am angry with_____for____

_____

_____

Once you have acknowledged what your anger is about, the next step is finding ways to express it. Here are some suggestions. Feel free to add to the list.

Ways to Express Anger:

1. Hit a pillow—over and over again.
2. Sit in your car with the windows rolled up and scream.
3. Dance wildly.
4. Growl.
5. Write a letter to the person you are angry with; after it's done, you can decide whether you want to send it.
6. Chop wood; hammer nails.
7. Cry.
8. Stamp your feet; wave your hands.
9. Talk to a therapist about it; with his/her support, do a role play with the person with whom you are angry.
10. Say it directly.

11. _____

12. _____

13. _____

14. _____

Exercise 73: All My Anger

We often have distorted images of our anger. If we haven't given ourselves permission to express it for a long time, we tell ourselves that we can't begin now because if we did, we would explode or blow someone away or cause a tornado right there in our own houses.

Complete the sentence:
I'm afraid that if I let my anger out . . .

1. _____

2. _____

3. _____

4. _____

Remember that these are *fears*. Acknowledge them as such and then notice what happens when you really do express your anger in the moment.

Exercise 74: Unexpressed Anger

Complete the following sentences:

1. In the recent past, I felt angry with_____

about_____

_____

2. I didn't express it because_____

_____

3. What did you do with the anger?
Circle the appropriate answers:

I pushed it away.

Nothing.

I turned it against myself (i.e., by eating, drinking, etc.).

I turned it against my child (my friend, my lover, etc.).

I apologized.

I went to sleep.

4. After you did the above, how did you feel about the person with whom you were angry?

EXAMPLES:
a. I felt that I never wanted to see him again.
b. I felt distant from her.
Complete the sentence:
When I didn't express my anger with _____

I felt _____
about her/him.
5. How did you feel about yourself?

EXAMPLES:
a. I felt numb.
b. I felt ashamed of myself for being emotional and needing so much.

Complete the sentence:
When I didn't express my anger with _____, I felt

_____
about myself.

Exercise 75: Expressed Anger

Complete the following sentences:

1. In the recent past, I felt angry with_____

about_____

_____

_____

2. This is how I expressed it:

_____

_____

_____

3. After I expressed my anger, I felt:
   Circle the appropriate answers:

   relieved   sad   powerful

   satisfied   exposed   hurt

   cleansed   seen   proud

   angrier   complete   unfinished

4. This is how I felt about the person with whom I was angry:
   Some examples may be: I felt as if I could trust her/him because I knew that I could trust myself to take care of myself; I felt distant from her/him; I felt understood.

_____

_____

CHAPTER 13

Taking Care

Compulsive eating is an attempt to nourish ourselves physically, but it is only a symptom of our need to be nourished emotionally. Learning how to nourish ourselves in ways that don't involve food requires thought and a willingness to please ourselves, to treat ourselves the way we would treat someone we loved very much.

Exercise 76: Ways to Nourish Myself with Something Other Than Food

When we started using food to express our feelings, it was because no other resources were available to us. Food was convenient and fast and it tasted good. Now, however, we have other choices. When we are hungry, we can, of course, eat. But when we are not hungry, we can do a variety of other things as well.

When I ask workshop participants what they can do to nourish themselves besides eat, they often look at me blankly. They say, "There *is* nothing besides food!" When you have used food to comfort and protect you for years, it may seem as if there is nothing else that "does it as good." Discovering new ways to care for yourselves requires time, creativity, and practice.

If you didn't eat to comfort yourself, what would you do?

Complete the sentence:
Ways in which I can nourish myself without eating are:

129

EXAMPLES
1) Taking naps
2) Allowing myself to do nothing
3) Asking a friend to tell me three reasons why she likes me

1. _____

2. _____

3. _____

4. _____

5. _____

6. _____

7. _____

You could transfer this list to a large piece of paper and post it on your refrigerator. The next time you reach for food when you aren't hungry, you'll be reminded of other ways to take care of yourself.

Setting Limits and Practicing as Ways to Nourish Yourself

When you're doing something that doesn't feel good to you—i.e., eating when you are not hungry—you have these choices: You can continue to do it and not think about it; you can continue to do it and be aware of what you are doing; or you can make a decision to stop.

There is a fine line between judging yourself and stopping because you are bad and making a commitment to yourself and stopping in order to take care of yourself.

If I like sugary foods (and I do!) but notice that when I eat them I don't feel well afterward, my choice not to eat them comes from my desire to take care of myself, not deprive myself.

At some point—and you decide when that point is—you make a decision to stop doing what doesn't feel good. At first, you *practice* your decision, like practicing a musical instrument. In the beginning, you make a lot of mistakes. But you keep practicing. Making the decision to practice is a way of setting limits.

Another way of setting limits is by making a decision that, for instance, this week you will follow one of the seven Eating Guidelines every day. When you notice yourself not following it, you will begin following it.

It's very important to go as slowly as you need to go. If you decide to make too many changes all at once, you will get frustrated when you do it "wrong" and you will feel like a failure. To avoid the pain of failure, you might decide that you don't want to make *any* changes.

But when you *do* make a decision to practice something new, gently notice each time that you avoid doing it, and then begin practicing again. Eventually, all the eating guidelines and the loving ways you care for yourself will become effortless. You won't remember when you struggled so. But it takes great effort to be effortless.

Exercise 77: Setting Limits This Week

This week, I can practice taking care of myself with food by deciding to set certain limits. Some examples may be: setting down my fork every time I realize I feel satisfied; following one eating guide line every day. I can:

1. _____

_____

2. _____

_____

Saying No

Another way to take care of ourselves by setting limits is to say no. Most compulsive eaters are wonderful at nurturing others and not wonderful at nurturing themselves. In fact, "not nurturing" is a mild way of saying that for the most part, if we are compulsive about food, we simply do not know how to nurture ourselves. We don't believe we *deserve* to nurture ourselves; we *do* believe that if we stop taking such good care of others and begin taking care of ourselves, we might lose those we love. Or something else will fall apart.

We need to teach ourselves to care for ourselves. And one very essential way to do that is to learn to say no. "No, I don't want to do that right now"; "No, tonight is my night for myself and I promised myself I wouldn't make any other plans"; "No, I will not turn myself inside out so that you will love me"; "No."

If we feel that we're unlovable, and most of us do, then we often feel that we need to do things we really don't *want* to do to be loved. The net result, however, is that if we're doing things we don't really want to be doing, or giving things we don't really want to be giving, then we won't feel loved, anyway. We'll feel as if we are not being seen for who we are and that the love, therefore, is fake.

Today is a perfect day to begin saying no and to notice that the world doesn't crumble when you do. Sometimes saying no to someone else is saying yes to yourself.

Exercise 78: Saying No

To make this exercise safe, consider telling a friend that you are practicing saying no; ask her if she would like to practice, too. For the next month, allow yourself to say no to each other once a week. They can be very simple no's: "No, I don't want to take a walk right now"; "No, I don't want to eat at that restaurant again." Start with easy no's. After a while, you will feel more comfortable saying no and can begin practicing with bigger no's— no's that have to do with deep feelings, no's that have to do with not allowing yourself to be violated in any way.

This month, I said no to:

1. _____about_____

_____

2. _____about_____

_____

3. _____about_____

_____

4. _____about_____

_____

A bigger no that I want to say but have not yet said is_____

_____

The Other Side of No: Treating Your Body With Kindness

In the same way that we respond openly to loving words, our bodies respond to kindness. A few months ago, I realized that every single day when I awoke, I felt my stomach to see if it was big or little. If I felt it was too big, I sighed, disgusted with it. The message I was giving it was: "Oh, come on. Can't you get it together and be attractive? The way you are is big, fleshy, ugly."

My stomach is part of me. This was *me* I was talking to. This was *me* I was describing as ugly. And each time I did, the vulnerable part of me cringed. The criticism, of course, did nothing to change the shape of my stomach.

Our bodies are part of us. Just as we learn to treat ourselves with kindness, we must learn to treat our bodies lovingly. They've put up with a lot of abuse from us—we've starved them, overfed them—and they still continue to function.

Exercise 79: Mirror Work

This exercise will take a total of twenty minutes, spread over four days.

Go to a full-length mirror in your house. If you don't have

one, buy one. It's time you saw yourself from the neck down! And while you're standing there, read the following:

Day 1: For five minutes, just look at yourself with all your clothes on. Every time a negative judgment comes up, replace it with an observation. For instance: "Look at the ways my arms bulge" gets replaced with "As the line of my arms changes, it curves nicely in some places." Notice your eyes, your hair, your skin. Notice how lovely you are.

Day 2: Take the clothes off the top half of your body. For five minutes, watch all the judgments that arise and replace each one of them with an observation. Pay yourself one compliment.

Day 3: Take all your clothes off, and for five minutes notice how you feel when you look at your body. What are the first thoughts that arise when you look at your legs? Your hips? Notice the lines of your body, where it curves. Notice the texture of your skin. Replace every negative judgment with an observation. Pay yourself two compliments.

Day 4: Again, with no clothes on and for five minutes, look at yourself with an artist's eye. Are you round? Where? Are you fleshy? Where? *No* judgments. Appreciate this body for carrying you this far. Pay yourself three compliments.

After you are finished, answer the following:

1. The hardest thing about doing this exercise was_____

_____.

2. When I replaced the judgments with observations, I_____

_____

_____.

3. With an artist's eye, my body looks_____

_____.

4. Three compliments I paid myself are:

a. _____

b. _____

c. _____

Exercise 80: Body Parts*

On the following pages are two drawings: one of the front part of a body and the other of the back part.

You will need three crayons to complete this exercise.

1. With the first crayon, color the parts of your body that you don't like.
2. With the second crayon, color the parts of your body that you do like.
3. With the third crayon, color the parts of your body that you feel neutral about.
4. Pick an area of your body that you find disagreeable, an area that you find yourself constantly judging.
5. Complete the following sentences:

I am _____'s [your name] _____ [body part].

She/he usually tells me that I am_____

_____

and that I am_____

_____.

I need instead for her/him to_____

_____.

_____

*This exercise was designed by Amy Pine, a body-movement therapist in Santa Cruz.

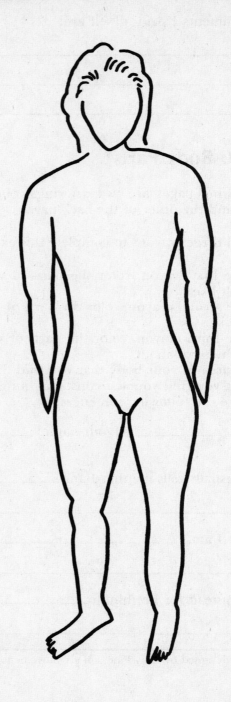

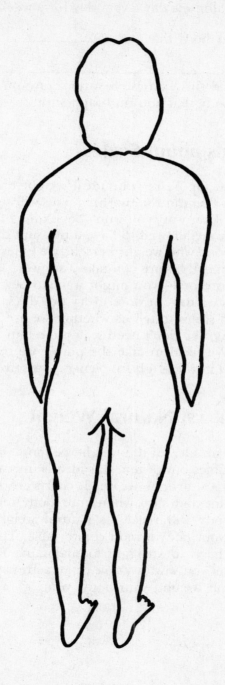

6. For one minute a day, every day for a week, I will tell this

   part of my body that_____

   _____

7. If you find this exercise helpful, move on to other parts
   of your body that you find fault with.

A Few Words about Scales

Throw them out. Or paste your ideal weight on them so that
when you get on them in the morning, you will see exactly what
you want to see. That way, you won't be asking a lifeless piece of
machinery if you are allowed to have a pleasant day.

If you're someone who weighs herself five times a day—before
you eat, after you eat, before you take a shower, after you take a
shower, and before bed—you might want to begin by weighing
yourself only once a day, or once every two days.

We don't need scales to tell us whether we are allowed to like
ourselves that day. We don't need scales to tell us if we've lost or
gained weight. We need to take the power we have invested in
scales and return it to its rightful owner—ourselves.

Ideal Weight vs. Natural Weight

We usually have an idea of the weight we most want to be—and
maintain. Nine times out of ten, this idea is unrealistic. It comes
from media images, articles we read, charts we see. When you
eat what you want and stop when your body tells you it's had
enough, your body will reach its natural weight. This is the
weight at which your body is most comfortable. This is the weight
that you don't have to struggle to maintain. This is not the
weight of a model you saw in *Vogue* or an actress you saw on the
screen; this is your weight, your body, you.

Exercise 81: Asking for What You Need

The hard part.

It's easy to give, harder to receive—and even harder to *ask* to receive.

What do you do when it's time to ask for what you need or want?

EXAMPLES:
1) I don't.
2) I have to be in serious trouble before I ask.
3) I feel that if I have to ask, it's not worth getting. Whoever I have to ask should know what I need without my saying so.

Complete the sentence:
When I need or want to ask for something, I:

1. _____

_____

2. _____

_____

3. _____

_____

4. _____

_____

Make a list of three things you wanted to ask for this week and didn't:

1. _____

_____

2. _____

_____

3. _____

_____

Make a list of three things you would like to ask for on a regular basis in your life:

EXAMPLES:
1) physical affection
2) time alone

1. _____

_____

2. _____

_____

3. _____

_____

This week, ask for two things. After you've asked for them, write them down.

Complete the following sentences:

1. I asked for_____

from_____. When I asked, I felt

_____

The response I received was_____

_____

2. I asked for_____from

_____. When I asked, I felt_____

_____. The

response I received was_____

_____

Asking and Receiving

It would be wonderful if, each time we asked, we received what
we asked for. The chances are that most of the time, we *will*
receive it. But there are bound to be times when we don't.

For many years, I wouldn't ask for anything if I thought there
was any possibility that the answer would be no. And, if I dared
to ask, I'd first try to guess the mood of the person I was asking
so that I could catch her or him feeling good and thus diminish
my chances of hearing "no." Sometimes I find myself still doing
this.

Asking is difficult because it makes us vulnerable. In asking,
we are saying, "I can't do it myself. I'd like you to help me. Will
you?" If someone says no, we often hear, "I don't love you"
rather than, "This is not a good time for me." If, every time we
ask, we feel we might hear that we aren't loved, we won't ever
ask.

There is another way, however, to ask. And that is, with the
realization that what we are truly saying is *"I am worth so much to
myself that I am willing to take a risk and ask for what I need."* Then if
someone says no, we are not crushed. They have not taken
anything from us. We began with the belief that we were lovable;
we are not dependent on someone to prove that to us. Asking
becomes what it is: an expression that we do not live in this
world alone. We need each other.

CHAPTER 14

In Favor of Support

The Breaking Free approach to compulsive eating is radical; most people believe that dieting or depriving themselves of certain foods is the only way to lose weight and end the obsession with food. Eating what you want when you are hungry and learning to nourish yourself in ways that don't involve food can be very lonely if everyone around you thinks you're crazy. You begin to doubt yourself, feel confused, and within a short time, believe that they are right: you *are* crazy. Don't allow yourself to be surrounded by people who don't understand or who want you to do what they are doing; find a network of support and if you can't find one, create one. It makes all the difference in the world.

And in your eating.

Gathering Together: Forming a Support Group

Beginning

You can start a self-led support group with a minimum of five people. Ten participants is ideal, twelve is maximum, but in my experience, you need at least five, including yourself, to feel as though you are actually in a group with direction and purpose, instead of meeting at someone's house for tea.

Spread the word in your community. Tell your friends what you want to do, talk to them about how they may be using food

142

in their lives. If you can't find enough people for a quorum, put an ad in the local paper that states the purpose of the group.

Place

When your group meets for the first time, decide on a single location at which every meeting will take place: someone's home, a community center, a women's center. Any place that will afford privacy and quiet, away from telephones, children, desks, and demands will do.

Time Commitment

I recommend that the members of the group make a commitment to meet for eight, ten, or twelve weeks. It is important to have a block of time together to develop trust, bonding, and a group rhythm. At the end of those weeks, the time commitment can be renegotiated.

Decide on the hours of the group during the first session. I recommend meeting for one and a half to two and a half hours each time.

Leadership

At the first meeting, decide whether you, as a group, are comfortable with rotating leadership—a different person leading the group each week—or one leader mutually decided upon. The task of the leader is to assign exercises to do at home, decide which exercises to do during the meeting, pay attention to time, and be certain that everyone gets a chance to speak.

Format

The session should be structured and purposeful, allowing space for people to share feelings, to recall incidents, to talk about what happened during the past week—as well as to focus and work together on a specific issue.

When a session begins, all members should be allotted three to five *uninterrupted* minutes to share about themselves, their feelings, their ongoing conflicts with food, their accomplishments during the week. (During the first meeting, this time can be used for introductions and weight histories). After each person has talked, time can be allotted specifically for feedback, encouragement, suggestions. Next, I suggest that you discuss the exercises that everyone did at home: problems, depressions, joys, questions.

The second half of the meeting can be devoted to doing an exercise from *Why Weight?*, *Breaking Free*, or other non-diet books you like. *Fat Is a Feminist Issue II* by Susie Orbach (Berkley, 1982) contains guided visualizations that I find provocative and useful. After the exercise or fantasy is complete, members can break into twosomes or small groups, to give everyone ample time to discuss her experience.

A self-led support group is not a therapy group. Some support groups find it helpful to have a therapist on call. They pay a therapist to attend one or two meetings so that participants who would like to work with a skilled practitioner in the framework of the group can have that opportunity. The therapist can also facilitate the resolution of problems that have arisen, make suggestions about specific issues, and observe and provide feedback about group dynamics.

Note: This is only an option; many groups do beautifully without it.

The Value of Therapy

I have been in therapy three times in my life. The first was when I was nineteen and my parents were getting divorced. The second was when I was twenty-seven and had gained fifty-five pounds. The third time is now.

When my first book, *Feeding the Hungry Heart*, was published, my former therapist called and asked why I hadn't written about the two and a half years I spent in therapy. I hesitated and then said that I hadn't wanted people to know. It was embarrassing, I said, to admit that I needed help to change old patterns. After all, we are supposed to be able to learn, to integrate, to grow, to accomplish, to become—on our own. Like normal people.

There is nothing "wrong" with being in therapy. While our culture defines therapy as something you seek out when you are disturbed—weak, sick, or crazy—I regard therapy as a way of moving closer to a vision of yourself in which you are connected to others and are fully alive. What could be disturbed about that?

The word "therapy" derives from a Greek word that connotes comrades in a common struggle. We *all* struggle to live richer, fuller lives. Depending on the environment in which we grew as children, depending on the permission we were given to express our sadness, loneliness, anger, to define our limits, we all struggle against the messages we received then that we now define as *truths*: We don't deserve to be happy; we need too much; we are selfish, we are mean. We are too intense. We are not lovable.

If we are remarkably fortunate or remarkably wise, we will know as adults that we are lovable, despite what we learned as children. If we are remarkably fortunate or remarkably wise, we will always draw people to us who see beyond our fears and protections, people who can stay with us without the fear of being destroyed, as we journey back to the point at which our vulnerability began. Although it might be true that therapy would be a waste of time for someone with this kind of fortune or this kind of wisdom, it is also true that in nine years of leading workshops and thirty-seven years of being alive, I have never met anyone who possessed this kind of fortune or this kind of wisdom.

At the end of every Breaking Free workshop, I talk about the importance of support. And I talk about therapy. Many participants have never had the experience of being in therapy and do not see how they might profit by it.

People go into therapy for different reasons. Some seek a therapist because they want to work on a particular problem; others begin therapy because they feel vaguely dissatisfied with their lives; still others begin because they don't like waking up day after day. When I began therapy this last time, it was because I saw myself repeating a particular pattern in my closest relationships; I heard myself saying "go away a little closer." I wanted to change that, I wanted to explore, to re-experience why I made the decisions I did about love—and I wanted to heal.

The frequency of visits (once a week, twice a week, once a month) and the length of time actually spent in therapy—whether it be six months or several years—is completely individual and depends on such fine factors as what you need and such coarse factors as how much money you can afford to spend on getting what you need.

The first step is often the most difficult: deciding that you want to *begin.* It is difficult because it means acknowledging—not avoiding—the fact that something is keeping you from living at the depth and with the joy that you sense is possible. Whatever that something is, you and those around you might be so close to it that you can't see your way clear without outside help.

Once you recognize the wish or the need for a therapist, you have to find one, and that step can take anywhere from two weeks to two years. I say this because I know; it took an entire year to find the therapist I am now seeing.

At first I told myself that because Santa Cruz is a small town and I knew all the therapists, I couldn't possibly begin treatment because I didn't want to see anyone I already knew. When I finally called a few of the therapists I did know and asked them for some referrals, I waited weeks to contact the people whose names I'd been given. Then, if a therapist I phoned did not return my call immediately, I began creating scenarios about being in a crisis, needing to talk to her or him and not having my call returned. When my phone calls actually were returned and I was on the other end of the line with a person (and not just an idea), I fumbled and stuttered my way through the conversation. "Hi. I got your name from _____. I, uh, I was thinking maybe I would like to come in and talk with you. I have been having, uh, yeah well anyway, I have been having problems with my, uh, relationships and I think I could use some [this next word was the hardest to get out of my mouth]—help." At this point in the conversation, although only seconds might have passed, I would feel I had made a fool of myself, that it was taking too long for the therapist to whom I was talking to respond and that the whole notion of therapy was ridiculous. Because I couldn't say, "Talking to you has made me realize that I am much healthier than I thought and so thank you for calling me back but I don't need the therapy," I would make an appointment for a session the following week.

Looking back on that time, I see that although I thought I had made a firm decision to begin therapy, I was still ambivalent and self-conscious about it. I dragged myself to the appointments I made—unless I cancelled them first. Choosing a therapist involves not only shopping around to find someone you truly feel seen by, but being willing to accept the vision of yourself as someone who asks for help because she cares enough about herself to take the time to find it.

In selecting one therapist over another, it is important to be aware of what your needs are—and to know that you have a right to choose whoever might help you. Some people want or need a therapist who is confrontative—a strong personality, someone who will actively seek them out when they are hiding. Others need a therapist who plays a quieter role, a person who listens and adds her or his observations at key moments in the session. There are different schools of therapy, different models of practicing it. It may not be crucial for you to know the model your therapist uses (unless, of course, you want to know and then all you have to do is ask), but it is important for you to know what, in a relationship, allows you to feel cared about and seen.

Maybe you don't know. Maybe you've never felt cared about in a way that satisfied your hunger to be seen and loved and so you don't know what to look for or what to ask for. You don't know if it's possible to receive what you've never received. It is not too late to find out.

You can begin by asking yourself what you longed for—and didn't receive—as a child. Were you listened to? Were you taken seriously? Were you allowed to express your anger, sadness, frustration, pain? Did your family try to talk you out of your feelings? And what about your present life—by whom do you feel loved? What are you receiving from them that you translate as love? Is it acceptance, patience, a willingness to stay with you when you are sad or angry? What is missing from your relationships?

I interviewed three therapists this time. The first, a woman in her sixties, had been trained as a Jungian analyst and emphasized dream work. I liked the fact that she was much older than I and had already experienced the years of life that were just beginning for me; I believed that she could offer me wisdom I couldn't get by working with someone closer to my own age. But as the session moved on, I felt as if she was leaving me behind. I didn't follow or necessarily believe her interpretation of my dreams. I left her office with an uneasy sense of having missed a connection with her. Later I realized that it was she who had missed making a connection with me.

The second therapist was a man, a psychiatrist highly recommended by other therapists in town. Two friends were seeing him regularly and reported him to be brilliant, sensitive, and compassionate, all of which I might have been able to see had I not wanted to crawl under the couch in his office. He responded to me with a kind of fierce intensity that made me feel very small and negatively judged. "If you want your entire experience to be about learning how not to be intimidated by him," said my friend Sara, "then by all means see him as a therapist." I decided that I had more pressing things to work on—like how I loved and let myself be loved. Cancel therapist #2.

It took three sessions of seeing #3 before I decided to begin therapy with her. It took three sessions because I wanted to be enthralled. I wanted to walk into a room, take one look at my therapist-to-be and *know* that she was the one. I wanted a therapist in shining armor. I wanted her to sweep me off my feet, to lock her eyes with mine, to make it impossible for me not to come back. She didn't. She was soft, she was gentle, but she left me with the responsibility of committing myself to working with her. I didn't like that.

When I called to cancel my third appointment with her, she remarked that if it was intimacy I wanted to work on, I couldn't do it by creating distance. There was no judgment in her voice; she said nothing that made me want to rise and defend myself. I felt *seen* by her, I felt cared about, and I felt the space—and responsibility—to decide if I wanted to do something different about my life. I decided that I did. I kept my appointment with her the following week. And the week after that. And the week after that.

A therapist becomes a loving parent, a best friend, and neither of the two. In the best of therapy, a therapist is someone by whom you feel valued and understood and with whom you are willing to explore the edges of yourself, the places you would not venture to go alone. Being in therapy, when it is working, allows you to reexperience the vulnerability of the child you were and re-evaluate the beliefs you formed about loving and being loved.

Being in therapy allows you to experience old beginnings—your pain, your fear—with new endings. When one person, a therapist, responds to you with thoughtfulness and compassion, by truly listening to you, valuing you, and seeing what you know to be true about yourself but cannot yet act on; when this one person is not afraid of your pain or intensity, but meets you where you weren't sure anyone could reach—the experience is yours to keep. And if that experience is possible with one person, even someone for whose time you are paying, it becomes possible with another. And another. Healing begins with the respect and care you learn for yourself in therapy and continues when you realize that what you feel *in* therapy is possible *outside* of therapy. Such an understanding is reached by those who are remarkably fortunate or remarkably wise. Or both.

Choosing a Therapist

- Ask your friends for names of respected therapists whom they have either heard of or with whom they have been in therapy.
- If you feel strongly about seeing either a woman or a man, respect that conviction. Although I have never been in therapy with a man on a long-term basis, I believe that a sensitive human being is a sensitive human being, man or woman. If you don't know how to decide, talk to therapists of both genders and notice your feelings. A decision depends on the particular man, the particular woman.
- If you are looking for a therapist who is sensitive to eating disorders and who deals with his/her clients in a non-deprivational way, call your local women's center and ask if they know anyone to whom they can refer you.

- Give yourself permission to shop around. Call a few therapists and tell them the truth—that you are in the process of looking and would like to meet them for a decisive session.
- When you are interviewing a therapist, remember that you can ask all that you want to know about how she or he* deals with clients. If you want to work on food and body image, ask her to tell you what she thinks about dieting. Ask if she has ever had an eating disorder. If so, what did she do to heal herself? If she has never had an eating disorder, has she read *Fat Is a Feminist Issue* (Berkley, 1978), *Feeding the Hungry Heart* (Signet, 1980), *Breaking Free* (Signet, 1986), *The Obsession* (Harper & Row, 1981)? If she hasn't, is she willing to? Tell her about this workbook and ask if following it is compatible with her beliefs.
- Notice how you feel about being in close quarters with this person. Are you reassured by looking at her face? Do you like her smile? (These questions are not on a list of essential things to consider in choosing a therapist, but you will be spending many hours with this person and it helps if you like being in her presence.)
- Be aware of the qualities you respect in others, qualities that put you at ease and allow you to feel safe. Know your own needs (if it's to be enthralled, maybe you should consider your needs again . . .). If you are contemplating therapy in order to deal with your weight and this particular therapist has never had an eating disorder or is herself fifty pounds heavier than her natural weight, you must assess what difference this makes to you. Some people feel comfortable with someone who shares their same problem, but is a little further along in her progress. Others would have a hard time respecting or believing in a therapist who hasn't resolved her own weight issues. No one can answer these questions for you.
- Trust what you feel when you are in her presence. Notice the nonverbal communication. Are you at ease? Is your stomach in knots, is your back tight? Do you feel accepted by her, do you feel judged? How does she deal with boundaries, limits, time constraints?
- When the session is over, does she tell you in a firm, gentle way—or do you feel she is letting your session spill into the

---

*For convenience, the pronoun "she" is used throughout these pages.

next hour? Being able to say no, establishing limits, taking care
of yourself are crucial issues in resolving compulsive eating.
Your therapist can be a model for you; in dealing with you, she
can teach you to do things you'd be frightened of doing alone.
- Notice her body language. Does she seem comfortable with
  herself? Is she open and affirming about sexuality? Is she
  homophobic? You can learn these answers by watching and
  asking her.
- How does she handle the question of money? What would
  happen if you didn't have the money to pay her one week?
  Does she have a sliding scale? Is she apologetic about what she
  charges or is she at ease with the value she places on her time?
- Finally, do you like her? Does she have a sense of humor?
  This business about living and growing can get too serious;
  sometimes you need to kick back your chair and laugh—and
  sometimes you need to kick back your chair and *guffaw*—at the
  silliness of it all.

After a Month of Seeing a Therapist . . .

How do you feel about the time you have spent with her? Are
you satisfied with the way she is responding to you? Do you feel
you are making progress inside yourself?

Although it may take much longer than a month to effect
major changes in your life, it takes only a willingness to be
honest with yourself now to decide how it feels to be face to face
with this person week after week, this person who is your therapist.

It is possible that even after careful decision making, there
may be something missing, something that isn't quite right about
your connection with her. Too often, the responsibility for this
not-quite-rightness is given to and accepted by the client—you.
You may feel you haven't been working hard enough. Or you
may feel a vague uneasiness about your time with her and blame
it on your neediness or your craziness or your intensity. If so,
evaluate your time with her. If you feel uneasy or disturbed
about it and/or yourself, talk about it in your next session. Tell
the truth. If you don't express your feelings because you are
afraid of hurting your therapist's feelings, you will be paying a

lot of money to perpetuate old patterns; your time in therapy will be wasted. Worse, you will feel even more isolated and alone than before you started therapy because now you will have added a new song to your already extensive catalogue of self-defeating tapes. This new tune is: You can't even do therapy right—there really is no hope.

Therapists are people, too. Not one of them is perfect, and some are less perfect than others. Or, as a friend of mine says, "Therapists are like hairdressers. There are some whose work deserves an 'A' and some who don't even earn a 'D.' It's not the technical training, because even a technically perfect haircut can leave the customer unhappy. The hairdresser has to know when to leave that corner alone. She has to know how to combine her expertise with her customer's needs—and if she doesn't know how to do that, nothing else really matters. And the customer should find another one because God knows, there are enough hairdressers around. Kind of like therapists."

CHAPTER 15

For Every Season . . .

Suggestions for Change During the Year

During each season, the light changes, the temperature changes, and we change. What we do, what we eat, what we wear, where we go—all change with the movement of the sun.

As you move through the seasons, compare my observations with your experience. Read through the suggestions on the following pages and make a commitment to yourself to do at least three of them during that particular season. Don't forget to enjoy yourself.

Winter

Winter. The frenzy of the holidays shrieks to an abrupt halt. The ground freezes, the sky is gray, the air is cold. Winter is like the space between breaths, the stretch of time in which the trees, the flowers, the earth are still.

How do you feel about winter? Do you miss the constant motion, the vibrant colors, the heat? I used to hate winter until I realized that I had a winter, too—and that the acres of muted colors and intense silence outside me reflected spirals of intense silence and colorlessness inside me. I used to hate winter until I began finding in it permission to not be vibrant all the time, to go inside, to be silent.

Sometimes in winter we can seem insignificant and situations can seem overwhelming. Bare trees, darkness at five P.M. Someone we love has just left. Given that seasons change, people leave, things change, things happen that are not in our control, the choice about how we act is sometimes the only choice we have.

Here are a few suggestions I have found helpful for staying warm and happy in winter:

- Be flexible about what you eat. Know that your body needs different foods in winter from the ones it needs in summer. Cold foods make you cold. Without thinking about calories, take a moment now to imagine what foods would feel best inside you tonight, tomorrow. How about hot, thick soups, biscuits, rice, vegetables (I'm devoted to butternut squash), beans, warm bread pudding. Not all in one day, of course. But then again, if you eat when you are hungry and stop when your body has had enough . . .
- Be flexible about what you do and the pace at which you do it. In the summer, for instance, I take four or five dance classes a week and spend a lot of time outside, going, doing at a fast pace. In the winter, my needs change. I like being indoors, and when I exercise, I like staying close to home. So instead of dancing, I'll walk or run. What about you? What kind of movement does your body want to go through in the winter? Don't be afraid to listen to it; it won't betray you.
- Find something luscious to do that doesn't involve food. If you like being outside in winter, organize a weekly get-together with friends and do what you love most. If you like being indoors, organize a weekly craft circle or reading-out-loud circle. Decide what you want in your life (i.e., closeness, outside sports, reliable contact, alone-time)—and then consciously structure your time so that you feel your life is rich and abundant.
- Get serious about something that you've always intended to take up but never have: playing a musical instrument, knitting, woodworking, writing, painting. And then there are always closets to clean.
- Remember that winter is absolutely always followed by spring.

Exercise 82: Winter and Me

Complete the following sentences:

1. I like winter because_____

_____

_____

2. I don't like winter because_____

_____

_____

3. I eat differently in winter because_____

_____

_____

4. Things I like to eat in winter are_____

_____

_____

5. My feelings about my body change in winter in these ways:

    a. _____

    b. _____

    c. _____

6. Three things I will do this winter to make myself feel good are:

a. _____

_____

b. _____

_____

c. _____

_____

Spring

When you make it through January and February, which always seem to be the darkest months of winter, spring and daffodils cannot be too far away. Spring spills along in bursts of color and light. Sometimes the quality of the light is so sharp, so gorgeous that you can't believe you are alive to see it. And sometimes, you get so caught up in day-to-day personal dramas that you forget to look. Don't live your life forgetting to look. Don't live a single day forgetting to look. You can choose.

It's spring.

It's time to:

- Spend five minutes a day listening to a bird sing.
- Notice the new green on trees, bushes, everywhere.
- Fill your house with flowers.
- Clean out your closet and give away any clothes that don't fit. This means all the pants and skirts you are waiting until you lose weight to fit into.
- Buy at least one new article of clothing in a color you could drink.

Summer

Summer days are long, longer, longest—and wildflowers are everywhere. Summer makes me want to play, pick honeysuckle, jump rope—be a kid again and take two months off from school. It's time for shorts and sleeveless tops, time for bathing suits, time for seeing bodies (everywhere—in the grocery store, on the beach, at the gas station) that are svelte and sleek and bare.

The coming of summer brings you the panic of bare thighs, and the thought of bare thighs may bring on hysteria. Only going on a diet—any diet, even hard-boiled-eggs-and-spinach, even prunes-and-meatballs—can alleviate your feelings about those bare thighs.

To prevent you from doing anything drastic, I want to remind you of a few details that you may be overlooking as it gets warm.

1. Chances are that this is not the last summer you will be alive. You will have many more opportunities to be svelte and sleek and bare, if that's what you really want.
2. Dieting solves nothing. It is nothing but a Band-Aid applied to a very deep wound.
3. If you go on a diet, there is a 98 percent chance that you will gain the weight back.
4. Hating the weight of your body does not make it go away.
5. Your thighs, your midriff, your arms are not as unattractive as you think they are.
6. If you eat when you are hungry, pay attention to the food, and stop when your body has had enough, you will lose weight.
7. Sleek, svelte, and bare bodies do not necessarily belong to happy hearts.
8. Mangoes, strawberries, and ice cream are infinitely more delicious than prunes and meatballs.

Instead of Dieting

1. Buy yourself a few pieces of summer clothing that fit you *now*. Buy them in luscious colors.
2. If your clothes can be luscious, so can the food you eat. But remember that what you want to eat is often different from what you think you should want or what you think you shouldn't want. Leave your mind out of the decision. What would make your body feel good? How do you want to feel when you finish eating? Your needs

and desires for food change with the seasons—how is what your body wants (when it is hungry, of course) different now from what it was in spring? In winter?

3. Do something wonderfully rewarding for yourself every single day. Take half an hour to go for a walk, dig a garden, read a book, practice the piano, take a nap. Something. You need to make it clear to yourself that despite the fact that you do not have a perfect body, you deserve to be joyful, absolutely delighted—even ecstatic—about being you, about being alive. It's summer—take in the beauties of the season. It'll be another year before you have the chance again.

Autumn

Fall may announce itself in crumpled leaves, or by the spontaneous yearning for fresh-pressed cider.

As fall begins you can:

- Walk in the leaves, crunching them underfoot. Jump in them—or press some between the pages of a book.
- Take advantage of the Jewish New Year by joining in the activities/festivities.
- Go to a fall festival you've never attended before.
- Register for a course at a local school.
- Visit an autumn exhibit at the museum.
- Go through last year's winter clothes and give away the ones that don't fit. Give away is not the same as putting them in the back of the closet and trying them on every week to see if they "fit yet."
- Pay close attention to the change in the weather and how it affects your body. In fall, our bodies generally need different kinds of foods than they did in summer. Warmer foods. More substantial foods. Be aware of getting stuck in summer food ruts or of being frightened to eat foods that have more calories than peaches and watermelons do.
- Play. Every day for at least fifteen minutes. Buy fingerpaints and make pictures. Buy body paints and paint someone else. Be the kid you are. It's okay to shout. And laugh.

CHAPTER 16

Making It Through the Holidays

Ah, the holidays. The impossible mixture of nostalgia for a childhood Chanukah or Christmas that may—or may not—have been real. The hope that this year will be different. The disappointment when it's not. And the food.

The food.

The connection between being happy and eating is probably stronger during the holidays than at any other time of the year. For many of us, being happy at Chanukah and Christmas is the same as eating with abandon. Something about the holidays only coming once a year. Something about working hard and deserving to celebrate. Something about assuaging a vague sense of bewilderment with what seems to be making everyone else happy: food.

When I talk to participants in Breaking Free workshops about their attempts at good cheer, most of them say that they handle food with a kind of recklessness, while masking an underlying sense of despair about the weight they know they must be gaining. They want to be happy. They want to have holidays of roasted chestnuts and open fires, but they feel overwhelmed by expectation and memories and instead of paying close attention to their needs and being gentle with themselves, they deal with their feelings by eating.

Whether they are alone and do not wish to be, or not alone and wish they were, their common problem is how to untangle themselves from the complicated web of nostalgia, feigned merriment, obligatory buying, and frantic eating to create a holiday in which they can enjoy the pleasures of the season without burying themselves in food.

Exercise 83: Holiday Fears

What are your fears during the holidays?

EXAMPLES:
1) I'm afraid that I will get into a painful argument with my mother.
2) I am afraid that I will eat pumpkin pies—whole.

When the holidays come, I'm afraid I will:

1. _____

_____

2. _____

_____

3. _____

_____

4. _____

_____

Exercise 84: On Being Alone

Complete the sentence:
If I am alone during the holidays, I will:

1. _____

_____

2. _____

_____

3. _____

_____

4. _____

Only _____ people are alone during the holidays:
Check the answers that apply:

       —desperate   —unhappy
       —unloved   —busy
       —self-satisfied   —self-confident

Exercise 85: Holiday Socializing

Complete the sentence:
If I spend time during the holidays with people I'm not truly
connected to, I will feel:

1. _____

2. _____

3. _____

4. _____

Exercise 86: Chanukahs and Christmases Past

It is important to separate the nostalgia for holidays past from
the reality of what is possible this year, this holiday, now. Because the holidays come once a year, we use them as marking
points to look back on the past and compare it with the present.
If, in the comparison, this year falls short of what we think is
possible (based on memories of holidays past), we become depressed or sad and are likely to turn to eggnog and fudge for
comfort. Yet our memories of a past holiday do not necessarily
reflect what actually happened during that holiday. For instance,
when I remember favorite holiday seasons, I see my father

taking my brother and me to see Santa Claus at the *Daily News* building. I see us telling him what we wanted, I see his beard, and I see him smiling and handing each of us a red helium balloon. That day is usually relegated to my category of "unequivocally happy times," and when I am feeling lonely during the holidays, recalling it makes me long for the kind of well-being I felt on Santa's lap, with my father and brother nearby. Now, as I write, and the details of that day become clear, I remember the fight my brother and I had about who had the best balloon and the tears that ensued when he put a pin in mine.

If a memory is perfectly happy, it is usually an indicator that we are remembering how we wanted it to be instead of the way it actually was. My image of a daddy taking his children to see Santa is colored by the perfection that is only possible with the passage of time. When we compare past holidays with the present and turn to food for comfort because the present lacks the love of the past, it is not because this holiday is so awful, but because we have warped the past into a time so flawless that it can never be achieved in the moment. This holiday can never be as good as the past one because the present is not—nor will it ever be—perfect.

Complete the sentences:
My perfect memories of Chanukahs or Christmases past include:

1. _____

_____

_____

_____

2. _____

_____

_____

3. _____

_____

_____

_____

4. _____

_____

_____

_____

If I didn't compare the holidays this year with memories in the past, I would:

EXAMPLES:
1) not decide that something was wrong with me because I am not part of a couple this year.
2) stop trying so hard to make each day a perfect day for my kids.

1. _____

_____

2. _____

_____

3. _____

_____

4. _____

_____

Being Realistic

The truth about holidays is that someone's balloon will always get a pin stuck in it. And that sometime during the six-week season, we are likely to be lonely or depressed. Not only because we are comparing the past with the present, but also because during any six weeks, we experience a broad range of emotions, some of which are happy and some of which are not. At Chanukah and Christmas, the expectation that we'll be happy and loving all the time is exaggerated by media images of cozy families, loving couples, and blissful reunions. No one reminds us that occasional misery is part of living from day to day, even in the midst of the season to be jolly. No room is provided for loneliness, no permission granted for sadness or depression, and when, inevitably, these feelings do arise, we use food to push them underground. If we can allow ourselves the expression of our feelings, we will not gain ten pounds in an attempt to bury them.

Is it possible, then, to have a happy and delicious holiday amidst unrealistic memories?

The answer is: yes, yes, a thousand times yes.

Exercise 87: Creating Happier Holidays

If you could have exactly what you wanted during the holidays, what would you have?

Complete the sentence:
For me, a happy holiday would mean:

EXAMPLES:
1) eating what I want when I am hungry and not overeating.
2) receiving only gifts that I like.
3) not having to go to parties when I'd rather stay home.

1. _____

2. _____

_____

3. _____

_____

4. _____

_____

Things I like best about the holidays are:

1. _____

2. _____

3. _____

4. _____

This year, I can include those things by:

1. _____

_____

2. _____

_____

3. _____

_____

4. _____

_____

The people I want to spend time with during the holidays are:

1. _____

2. _____

3. _____

4. _____

If I were my ideal weight this holiday season:
I would move . . .

EXAMPLE:
with grace and a swish.

1. _____

2. _____

3. _____

4. _____

I would talk . . .

EXAMPLE:
with ease.

1. _____

2. _____

3. _____

4. _____

I would eat/drink:

EXAMPLE:
Alta Dena honey eggnog.

1. _____

2. _____

3. _____

4. _____

I would act . . .

EXAMPLE:
as though I know I'm special.

1. _____

2. _____

3. _____

4. _____

Being aware of what happiness during the holidays means to you is the first step.

The next step is giving yourself permission to have it.

Additional Suggestions During the Holidays . . .

If You Are Alone

- Be aware that the holidays are promoted as a time of togetherness and love and that you are very susceptible to the belief that something is wrong with you because you don't have a lover. Nothing is wrong with you. Remind yourself that, as my mother once said, "Going to bed alone is lonely, but going to bed with someone who tears your heart out is worse." Congratulate yourself for not going to bed with someone who tears your heart out.
- Make contact with people you love. Write letters, send cards, make phone calls. Let yourself be filled with the love that is already in your life.
- Do something holiday-like for yourself every day, something you would ordinarily save for a time when you're with someone. Buy yourself a present. Set the table with holiday candles, decorate a plant with tinsel, drink eggnog from a champagne glass.
- If you know ahead of time that certain days trigger depression or loneliness or sadness, plan ahead. Be sure you take care of

yourself especially well at those times, either by being with friends and/or being in an environment that you find nourishing.

If You Are Returning Home

- Bring reminders of your present life—a journal, a tape, a favorite pillowcase, a cherished letter. Use them when you have forgotten that you ever left your parents' home.
- Do not expect to reenact holidays past. That was then and this is now. All of you have changed.
- Do, however, be aware of what made those holidays so special. If it was traditional family events, like playing with dreidels, eating potato latkes, or going to midnight mass, and it seems appropriate to continue the tradition, suggest that you do so. But if, for instance, a family member has developed an allergy to potatoes (or to mass) in the past few years, be creative about ways to be together. Remember that it's the sharing that's important and not the event that triggers it.
- Do not confuse receiving love with eating what was made in its name. You cannot eat love. If you are not hungry and food is placed in front of you, you can: Comment on how it looks and smells; ask about the ingredients; express your appreciation for the time it took to prepare the food; eat it when you are hungry.
- Eat exactly what you want when you are hungry. Give yourself permission to really enjoy what you eat. Do not solicit opinions from family members about how you look or what you eat; keep that power for yourself.
- Do something just for yourself every day. Spend some time alone. Remind yourself of your separateness. And your beauty.

Wherever You Are and Whomever You Are With

- If the holidays are particularly hectic for you, make a schedule for yourself. Decide which days you will shop and which days you will cook. Decide on a budget for gifts (and stick to it). Don't allow yourself to be the victim of last-minute panic. You really *can* have a relaxed season.
- Be conscious of food. Very, very, conscious. While holidays are not a time to deprive yourself—there is no time when depriv-

ing yourself is healthy or healing or works to your advantage—
neither are they a time to make yourself sick. If you like
homemade candy, eat it. If you like butter cookies, eat them.
But taste them, savor them—and stop when your body tells
you it has had enough. The attitude that "The holidays only
come once a year and this is my last change to eat _____
[fill in the blank] so I'd better eat all I can now" leads to
emotional and physical discomfort. It is not an attitude that's
based in reality. You can bake Christmas cookies in mid-April;
Hummantaschen in October; you can whip up homemade candy
at the beginning of June. Eating with abandon during the
holidays is not a way to have fun; it is a way to numb yourself
so that you never feel anything but alternately gleeful about how
much you are eating and miserable about how fat you are getting. When you knock yourself out with food, you never feel the
subtle but tender moments, the fleeting glances of intimacy,
the energy of the season, the excitement that has nothing to do
with food. You also never feel, and therefore can do nothing
about, your discomfort or bewilderment or dissatisfaction.

- Set aside some time for yourself every day. In the rush of the
holidays, we often forget to do the quiet things that nourish us.
We spend our time thinking about others (which is, admittedly,
a lovely thing to do) and have the tendency to forget to pay
attention to our own needs. When we feel depleted, and food
is as available as it is during the holidays, we use it to fill us. Go
for a motorcycle ride, begin a novel, sit in a chair and do
nothing. When you take time for yourself, you remind yourself
that you are worth taking time for.

- Make a list of the things you like most about the holidays. Do
at least one of them each day. Give yourself something to look
forward to, give yourself some power in creating a holiday
that is joyful to you.

- When you go to a party at which there is a buffet, take a
sampling of three dishes that look inviting to you. Take your
time eating them. Enjoy them. If you want more, take more
but do it slowly, savoring each bite so that you don't feel
sickened by the amount of food.

- Remember that you do not have to go to a party simply
because you are invited to it. Be aware that you have choices
about what to do with your time.

Taking care of yourself during the holidays means that when you are hungry for food, you eat with pleasure and gusto, savoring the tastes of the holidays. When you are hungry for something else—a touch, a word, a moment of contact, some time alone—taking care of yourself means being willing to ask for and receive those pleasures, those tastes of Chanukah and Christmas.

The holidays are the time when the sun begins to return to us, when the days become lighter and longer. They are the time when people are willing to put their ordinary concerns aside and spend their time giving, wishing for the best, thinking about peace. When I see, even for a moment, that people are capable of giving and bending and making peace, it makes me believe it is possible for another moment and another. For a whole string of moments, for a year. For the rest of our lives.

CHAPTER 17

Letters from the Journey

I receive many letters each week from people who are struggling with—and breaking free from—a lifetime of compulsive eating by following the guidelines in this book. For those of you who think that this method can work for me but not for you, or that your problems are different from or worse than anyone else's, or that I am a special case because of my history, age, commitment, etc., I have included a sampling of these letters to provide you with other voices and to let you know that you are not alone.

Dear Geneen,

Halfway through my dinner tonight I stopped—put my fork down and burst into a deep-seated cry that felt like unleashing a dam. I'm crying even as I write this, but who else could I tell a fourteen-year-old secret that revolves around food? The tears tonight and for the last two weeks have been out of happiness for the first time since I was twelve.

I am a twenty-six-year-old female who is an attractive and talented artist who has had bulimia since 1972. My father died of cancer at the age of thirty-four, leaving my alcoholic mother and three sisters to survive. I am the eldest, who decided after five years of psychotherapy that I was a lost cause and that trying to stop bingeing at this point was ridiculous. In the past, especially through college, my depression was severe and mostly brought on by the bulimia. I am not now and have never been overweight, but the guilt from bingeing has driven me so far into depths of myself that I can't remember ever feeling normal.

I recently was hospitalized for a spastic colon caused by stress. After being on an I.V. for eight days and having the very needed time to reflect on the past fourteen years without food there to numb me and distract me—I realized that it was now or never—maybe even literally. Either I stopped throwing up after every meal and stopped using laxatives, or the inside of me would simply give up one day and fall apart. So, I got out of the hospital and bought several books, one of which was *Feeding the Hungry Heart.*

It wasn't until I saw a TV show some weeks later that I really broke down and sobbed. Nothing in my life had changed—I cried out of fear and mostly desperation that I would and could *never* get a grip on my life. Two weeks later I bought another book, *Breaking Free from Compulsive Eating.*

Up until I purchased your book, my biggest challenge (and only now can I call it a challenge) was coming home from work to my house where I live alone. There have been two years of evenings where I have dreaded being able to eat anything I wanted. I just wasn't thinking then. I was caught in a struggle with myself that had lasted so long that I couldn't remember what it was about, so I guess that habit stepped in even when I didn't want to binge.

Two weeks ago, I broke a date on a Friday night to read your book. I was afraid that the book would either say nothing to me that I hadn't already heard or maybe it would say everything to me that I needed to hear. I have to tell you that I haven't finished it yet. Not because I am a slow reader, but I didn't really need to continue after chapter five and I think that part of me is afraid for it to end. Whatever, the combination of things you said had already taken their effect halfway through the book and I fell asleep knowing that something was about to change in my life. *Finally.*

The first day was glorious—the second was wonderful—the third was unbelievable—fourteen years without missing more than a weekend between binges and here I am two weeks later feeling clear (only a binger knows that "clear" feeling). I am full of emotion, not food. The last four nights I've cried before finishing my dinner without an appetite to finish because of the amount of energy I have spent during the day confronting my inner self and by the time I eat dinner, I am exhausted and feeling so terrific that I cry—releasing again.

The real test was at my mother's house two days ago. I left there with such anger in my heart and stomach. I drove home knowing what she aroused in me—how she always made me feel—full of anxiety. I cried again in the car and then at the front door. I allowed myself to feel angry and hurt. All those years without letting it out, there's no wonder I've been so teary. I was alone and I faced myself and what I felt and I hugged and comforted myself until I stopped feeling bad and the thought of food never entered my mind except when I thought how strange a time it would have been to eat—it was something I had done more than half of my life and now it seemed strange . . . I said to myself with a grin, "Judith, you're Breaking Free" . . . and it was right then that I think I felt happier than I've ever felt in my life.

It must be wonderful to have changed so many of us (the people who only need a little guidance to accept themselves and become whole). Thank you, Geneen, from all of me, even those parts that have been hiding since I was twelve. I know it will be a long haul, but I've started something great and there's no stopping me now.

Sincerely,
Judith Hollister
Stamford, Connecticut

Dear Geneen,

I was introduced to you and Breaking Free two years ago this November. I can't believe it's been two years already. I was introduced in a very loving and supportive way by a woman whose name is Irene. She is a therapist who does work with compulsive overeaters. She's my age, thirty-five, and has had her own personal issues with eating. We really connected and work well together. I have made tremendous progress with much time, patience, perseverance, and a couple of friends— and you, Geneen, and your workshops and books. I finally feel "Free." Since Omega I have experienced wonderful things;

like not being afraid of eating out, not being afraid of my favorite foods. Not being afraid that eating my favorite foods or eating out will make me fat or will lead to a binge; and not being afraid that the binge will never end. It feels good not to be starved or stuffed, it feels good not to deprive myself. It feels good to have choice, it feels good to eat what I like and not feel guilty. It feels good to like myself and not be obsessed with foods, diets, and scales. It's been hard work, but well worth it.

I love you,
Sue Bergeron
Enfield, Connecticut

Dear Geneen,

Since returning from your workshop in Portland, Maine, I have had this overwhelming urge to put my feelings on paper and send them to you. Should I stumble, falter, or seem overelated at times, please bear with me, for I have never written a letter like this.

I was referred to a therapist in August of 1986, by a medical doctor, as well as a certified nutritionist because they could not understand how a person could gain eleven pounds in three weeks (this was the gaining side of the yo-yo syndrome I have lived with for thirty-five of my fifty-nine years on earth). Never had there been a period in my married life that I was not on a diet. I have been the whole route: fad diets, speed, shots, plus many multicolored pills; running to and from doctors and diets; always living with low self-esteem and great guilt for my compulsive eating binges and extreme high and low mood swings.

My therapist became my friend, as well as my mentor. Through intensive therapy, she guided me to the point where I could see that there is a light at the end of the tunnel. She also introduced me to your books last November. I devoured *Feeding the Hungry Heart* and went on to *Breaking Free from Compulsive Eating*. I adapted them both as a Bible of sorts, and from that point on, everything for me became "ACCORDING TO THE WORD OF GENEEN." I began to put what I had read to use. For the very first time in thirty-five years, I truly enjoyed a strawberry ice cream sundae, and remember vividly savoring every mouthful. What a beautiful happening to rub my stomach afterward, and feel so satisfied with no pangs of remorse or guilt. My dieting friends, as well as others, thought I was crazy to give up my diets and scale-watching to follow your teachings. Sheer panic took over when I no longer hopped on and off the scale, and stopped counting calories. I pushed onward until suddenly, people were commenting on my weight loss, as well as my clothes hanging so loose.

Then it was June, 1987, and I had an appointment with my rheumatologist. Weigh-in was a must. Lo and behold, I had dropped thirty-five pounds somewhere along the way. The doctor was pleased and amazed. In answer to his asking, "How?" I proceeded to tell him about "The word according to Geneen," and the phrase I had coined myself, "Diet and defeat are synonymous in my mind." He loved my "diet and defeat" term, and asked if he could use it for others because this man's theory of weight control was, "If you eat ten candy bars per day, cut down to five."

The same scene was reenacted the following week, when my internist had the pleasure of witnessing my weight loss on his scale. He was from the old school of strict dieting, nutritionist referral, etc. I proudly explained to him who Geneen Roth was, and all that I had been doing.

My therapist told me you were coming to Maine, and gave me a copy of your workshop program plus a registration form. I could not contain my excitement. If working with your books, on my own, could do this much for me, I could only imagine all the horizons that would open up for me by attending a Breaking Free Workshop.

When you walked into the room for the first time, I had this great urge to wave and shout, "Hi, Geneen, Old Friend. It's me, Dorothy. I'm over here," because I had the advantage of friendship and intimacy on my part, toward you, for the past ten months. Great, fantastic, and superb are adjectives that continued to wash over me, as we progressed through your workshop.

One of the most emotional and moving experiences of my fifty-nine years of life was finding the lost, lonely child inside of me, and being able to comfort and embrace her. I want to shout it to the world, "It works! Look at me, I am living proof that one can truly succeed at 'Breaking Free'!"

I would like to end this "letter-turned-mini-novel" by testifying to the new "in control" me, that also gave up the compulsive habit of cigarette smoking (average of one-plus packs per day) this past August 28, 1987, and I feel great. However, this "kicking the habit" contributed to my slip back of getting on a scale again, due to a sudden weight gain caused by an excessive compulsive eating binge (replacing one bad habit with another). After noting a fifteen-pound weight gain, I immediately called upon "the word according to Geneen," and am happy to say that there has been a weight drop, but most important is the fact that I am back on track again, and no longer addicted to nicotine nor chained to a pack of cigarettes. Isn't it great! I still have a ways to go, but I am in no hurry to get there because it is so beautiful along the way now. How wonderful to eat and savor every delightful mouth of food that leads to the ultimate satisfied stomach—a feeling that one never knows as a compulsive eater.

THANKS!

> Dorothy A. Deluca
> Vancouver, British Columbia
> Canada

Dear Geneen,

My name is Pat, which rhymes with fat. As far back as I can remember, my brothers and sisters teased me and called me "Fat Pat." I believed I was fat and felt humiliated and enormous. Only recently have I looked at photographs of myself at six or seven years and seen a child of average weight with curly brown hair and green eyes.

I knew nothing of sibling rivalry or competition. I could not understand my feelings of never getting enough and blamed myself for wanting too much. It was not that my parents were incapable of giving nine children what they needed—it was that I was too needy.

By the time I was in the fourth grade I wore "chubby" sizes

and felt very self-conscious. In the sixth grade, my body began to change and my parents put me on my first diet. I failed at it, and I went on dieting for the next nineteen years.

After nineteen years of depriving myself and bingeing, I hated myself, felt I was a total failure, and was desperate. The event that changed my life was reading the book *Feeding the Hungry Heart*. It was a book to live by—I laughed, cried, cheered, and grieved. I felt horror and sympathy, and great release. It was the first time anyone had ever really said what it's like to be a compulsive eater.

I struggled with the idea of change, and then stopped my lifetime of dieting and bingeing. I threw out my bathroom scales and stopped putting myself through an agony made possible by the random numbers that would appear as I slowly put my weight onto the scale. I realized that whether the number was 100 or 200 was unimportant, what mattered was that if it was more than I thought it should be, I was depressed. And, if it was less than I feared it would be, I was happy.

My greatest fear was that as soon as I stopped dieting I would gain a hundred pounds. I began to buy and eat foods I had not eaten in years. Every morning I would stand in front of the mirror without my clothes on and try to be gentle to myself. I tried to see myself without judgment, and slowly I began to sew my head and body together at the neck.

I stopped seeing food in terms of calorie counts and fat and began to eat what I wanted. Starting to acknowledge what food was doing for me, I stopped hating myself. When I stopped dieting, I stopped failing, and a vicious cycle that I never realized existed ceased.

I looked at my life, and decided that this was not a dress rehearsal, it was my only performance. I began to read every book about food, compulsions, and women that I could find. I started a journal and began to explore myself. What *had* food been doing for me?

The reasons for my eating began to make themselves known like nerve endings being exposed; I was in pain. The biggest thing that food had done for me was to numb me. It drew all of the blood to aid in digestion and allowed me to focus on the pain and fullness in my stomach, instead of the pain and emptiness that was my life.

Another thing that food did for me was to help stuff down and swallow a number of feelings that I had come to recognize as unacceptable. Feelings of anger, hate, pride, jealousy, and hurt. The food that I swallowed pushed the feelings into my greatest depths, and they stayed buried there for years.

The less concerned I became with my body size, the more concerned I became with my feelings. I forced myself to explore the depths of my inner self. It was there I had hidden so many emotions. In spite of great fear, one by one I explored each feeling, owned it, and got stronger.

A year later, I took stock of myself: I had not weighed myself in a year, had not been on a diet for a year, and had not gained or lost any weight, according to my clothes. I began to like myself.

I read *Breaking Free From Compulsive Eating* from cover to cover, trying to absorb it all at once. I was being as good to myself as I could be—but I still wanted to lose weight. I felt stuck in the third stage of Breaking Free, and I wanted to be in the fourth stage. I wanted to do more than read about breaking free—I wanted to experience it. So, I enrolled in a weekend workshop.

I flew in an airplane to a strange airport where there was no one to meet me, rented a car, drove through a mountain pass to Santa Cruz, and rented a motel room—all by myself, all for the first time in my life.

I got up the next morning and drove to the workshop and told my story to a group of twenty women of different ages and sizes who were all compulsive eaters. I listened to each of their stories and heard their pain, and I began to realize that the only way out of the pain was through it.

I wanted to skip the stage I was in, but it was really the key to what I needed. I needed to stay with the pain, to find more ways to nurture myself before I could come out of it. Pushing the pain aside with food had kept me from dealing with it, but it never got rid of it. I was afraid if I started crying I would not be able to stop.

The workshop was a safe place to talk and feel and experience in. Geneen, you were a great facilitator—you knew just what we were going through. I decided to try to find my natural signal for fullness the very next day, before the second session began. I had eaten about half of my breakfast when I suddenly sighed a long, deep sigh. I knew instinctively that I was full, and that if I continued to eat I would be eating compulsively. I put my fork down and pushed the plate away.

There was nothing on the plate that I could never have again when I got hungry. I felt a twinge of sadness as I watched the waitress disappear with it, but that dissolved when I remembered that I had finally found my "full" signal—a natural gentle sigh.

By the end of the two-day workshop, I felt sad to say good-bye to the friends I had made, the people I had touched, and their warmth. I had been bombarded with new thoughts and ideas, and I wondered how long it would all take to soak in. How would I change? How long would the reverberations of the experience continue?

It has been two and a half years since I first read *Feeding the Hungry Heart* and stopped dieting. One and a half years since the workshop. A year since I first decided to try waiting until I was hungry to eat Sunday brunch.

Taking myself to brunch was a treat I began to give myself, and I decided I would postpone it until I felt hungry. I went for a walk.

I walked out along the back bay waters and wildlife preserve. An occasional jogger passed me and the breeze ruffled through the reeds and my hair. The sky stretched away from me in endless blue, and the sandy bluffs kept the sun from my eyes.

The sandpipers chased the tide in and out while a blue heron silhouetted a graceful *S* against the seagrass. Ahead of me a cottontail sprang out and crossed my path. The songs of the meadowlarks and warblers surrounded me, and up above me a hawk circled.

I looked at my watch. It was one o'clock and I panicked. I was not hungry. What if I never got hungry again? I put my hand to my racing heart and laughed. Of course I would get hungry again, and then I could have whatever I wanted. Pancakes, or an omelette, or scrambled eggs with bacon and hashbrowns and a bagel with cream cheese.

I have learned to eat when I am hungry, and to stop when I am full. I overeat occasionally and I listen hard to hear what I am saying about it. Somewhere along the way I have gone down two sizes in my clothes. I have no idea how much I weigh, nor do I care.

Only recently have I discovered just what some foods do for me. When I am feeling angry, for example, I want something crunchy—an apple, or popcorn, or peanuts. When I feel sad I want something soothing, like chocolate ice cream. And when I feel lonely or empty, I want something substantial—a baked potato or a bowl of rice.

The reverberations are still coming down around my spiral of psychic growth, spurred on by the workshop. I continue to be good to myself, and to find new ways to take care of myself. I still write in my journal, and I take long walks and long baths, and I have gone back to school. I take myself to dinner, to movies, and to plays. I buy flowers for myself.

I like myself, and I have come to realize I am a nice person— intelligent, sensitive, honest, humorous, strong and courageous no matter how much I weigh. Now I can start to work on the important things, the things that really matter. It is good to break free—to be out and free at last.

Pat Fox
Seattle, Washington

CHAPTER 18

Questions and Answers

During the course of the workshops, and in response to newsletter articles, I am asked many questions. Here are some that are asked again and again.

QUESTION: I need more clarification about eating without distractions, especially reading while eating, which I love to do. What if you just don't have any other time to read?

ANSWER: There once was a Zen master who told his students, "When you read you should read and when you eat you should eat." They followed his teachings scupulously until they noticed that each morning at breakfast, he read the newspaper. Finally, one of his students approached him and said, "Master, you tell us that when we read we should read and when we eat we should eat, but we notice that when you eat, you read." And the master replied, "That's right. When you read, read, and when you eat, eat. But when you read and eat, read and eat."

The purpose of the eating guidelines is to heighten your enjoyment of food and to help you stay aware of each aspect of the eating experience, from the texture and taste of the food itself to the different sensations in your body as you move from hunger to satisfaction. If, after you experiment with eating without distractions, you discover that your enjoyment of food is considerably lessened—that you just can't enjoy a meal without a book or magazine in hand—then by all means, do what you enjoy: Eat and read.

If, however, you only have *time* to eat or read, and you don't have time to do both, then you need to look at how you are structuring your days. You are not allowing enough time for pleasure. You need some time during each day when you don't do anything—when you're not eating, or reading, but just relaxing with yourself. And you also need some time when you're actively enjoying yourself—reading, drawing, singing.

We are all so achievement-oriented. We rush around so much of the time that unless we're doing, doing, doing, we don't feel good about ourselves. It's very important to slow down, perhaps do less, but feel better about what we do.

QUESTION: You say I should eat what I want, but I'm a diabetic and some foods would really harm me. Does that mean Breaking Free is not for me?

ANSWER: A lot of people are hypoglycemic, diabetic, allergic or food-intolerant. What I tell these people is that taking care of yourself is the principal issue here. Eating what you want when you're hungry and stopping when you've had enough doesn't mean disregarding safety. If you're diabetic and eating two pints of ice cream sends you into insulin shock, that's not taking good care of yourself.

There are different levels of deprivation. There's the deprivation of "I can't have sugar or cookies because I'm diabetic," which is different from the deprivation of feeling sick after eating them. What you deprive yourself of then is allowing yourself to feel good. It's important for you to examine why it is you would want to eat something that you know isn't going to agree with you. There's a basic disharmony in that. If you're gravitating toward something that's going to do you harm, then you're not feeling very good about yourself; you want to hurt yourself in some way. You need to examine why you want to punish yourself, not why you want to eat foods that you're not allowed to eat.

QUESTION: Is there hope that I can ever stop bingeing?

ANSWER: Absolutely. If you can *start* eating, you can stop. Learning how to stop takes practice and patience. It's important not to say to yourself, "I'm bingeing; this is really terrible; I'm going to gain five pounds; I'm a failure." But rather say, "I'm eating, and I'm eating frantically right now. How can I help myself?"

If you want to stop bingeing there are a few things you can do. You can put down your fork or spoon, stop the hand-to-mouth motion, and walk into another room. You can switch your attention to something else (a book, a person, music). But if you feel that you can't stop/don't want to stop, then don't. You will stop at some point. And when you do it is important to be gentle with yourself, and say, "O.K., what was going on?"

After a binge, wait to eat until you're hungry. The greatest danger of a binge is the chain reaction it sets off for the next few days or weeks. We don't gain twenty pounds from one binge. It's the progressive effect that paralyzes us.

QUESTION: Does the Breaking Free approach work for anorexics and bulimics?

ANSWER: Anorexia and bulimia are both types of compulsive eating; they are variations on the theme of using food for emotional reasons. *Why Weight?* is written primarily for overeaters, however, because I know the landscape of overeating best. I believe it is essential for anorexics and bulimics to get good-quality and compassionate therapeutic and medical care from people who are experts in these areas. While both of these eating disorders stem from emotional conflicts, the physical damage can be severe, and in some cases, life threatening, if the problems are left untreated. When you are destroying your health, it is difficult to focus on hunger and nourishment.

QUESTION: What was the first realization you had that made you want to change?

ANSWER: I think the very first thing was realizing that I was in pain. Realizing that something was going on inside me and I was eating because of it. I asked myself, "Is eating going to help the pain go away?" And the answer was no.

QUESTION: Does your approach apply to men as well as women?

ANSWER: Yes. Both men and women use food to express what they consider "unacceptable" feelings. It's more complex for a woman than for a man, because in our culture, a woman often equates her self-worth with her appearance, while a man usually defines himself by his work, achievements, athletic ability, and financial status. A man doesn't have the same *amount* of pressure, but I think when it gets down to it, we all eat for the same emotional reasons. Those of us who eat emotionally, eat because we're in pain—and that's universal.

QUESTION: What happens when I stop eating compulsively? Won't I start being compulsive about something else?

ANSWER: Only if you haven't actually acknowledged the root of your conflicts with food.

People who exchange one compulsion for another—alcoholism for compulsive eating or compulsive eating for compulsive shopping, for example—have not allowed themselves to explore the deep-seated reasons they became compulsive to begin with. As long as the purpose a compulsion is serving remains unconscious—i.e., protecting you from feeling the pain of your mother's death, or whatever—you will hold onto it for survival's sake and exchange one compulsion for another. Breaking free from compulsive eating means becoming aware of your underlying pain and feelings and learning that it is acceptable to express them directly.

QUESTION: What do I do when I feel like I've blown it and want to give up on the whole notion of eating what I want? Should I just go back on a diet?

ANSWER: No. No. No. At the moment you want to give up, remember how many other times you've had this same feeling. Then tell yourself you can handle this moment differently. You can say, "This is really hard, but I have to be patient with myself." Remind yourself that if you leave yourself here, too, you'll find yourself at this difficult juncture again. Why not move *through* it this time? Now's your chance.

Conclusion

"People say that what we're all seeking is a meaning for life. I
don't think that's what we're really seeking. I think that what
we're seeking is an experience of being alive, so that our life
experiences on the purely physical plane will have resonances
within our own innermost being and reality, so that we actually
feel the rapture of being alive. That's what it's all finally about . . ."
—Joseph Campbell
The Power of Myth (New York: Doubleday, 1988)

The rapture of being alive.

A few days ago, I watched a television special on breast cancer,
hosted by Jill Eikenberry, during which a number of women
(and one man) spoke of their feelings and experiences in dealing
with their disease. One woman said that when her doctor told
her she had cancer, she "howled at the moon." Another said she
actually hauled off and socked her doctor. A third woman said
that after her breast was removed, she hid her naked body from
her husband until he realized what she was doing and told her
that he wanted her never to hide again because he loved her.
She said that at that moment, she realized she had what she'd
always wanted: the experience of being utterly loved for who she
was, not for what she looked like.

Most of the people interviewed on this program said that
cancer had brought them closer to "the rapture of being alive."
One woman said that if she had to do it over again, if she was
given the choice of having or not having cancer, she would
choose to have the disease because of what it had taught her. She
declared that she was more alive now than she had been before
she got sick.

In a similar way, the process of breaking free from compulsive
eating is one in which you can use your conflicts with food to
bring you closer to the rapture of life. You are fortunate to have
this guide. If you listen to what it is saying, instead of spending
your time howling at the moon, you can unlayer yourself bit by

bit until you get to your core, the center of your being that holds your dreams, your vitality, your true voice. Compulsive eating can become your friend, directing you to what you have not recognized or accepted or expressed about what it is to be you, with your body, your feelings. In this sense, your compulsive eating can lead you to the source of your own power. If you face it directly, it will confront you with feelings about your childhood, your parents, your friends, your lovers, your children, your work. It will confront you with the love that is present or absent in your life. It will confront you with the truth.

When you begin listening to this truth of yours, when you begin treating yourself as someone who is worth listening to, when you begin taking care of your needs, you also create space within yourself to take care of other living things: people, animals, trees, the planet we inhabit.

The earth is at its most crucial point in history because we are on the verge of destroying it—as well as ourselves. Between the greenhouse effect, the hole in the ozone, the stripping of natural resources, the proliferation of garbage, dolphins being senselessly killed by tuna fishermen, and whales that are still being eaten by the Eskimos and the Japanese—we are rapidly making the planet uninhabitable.

And what is *outside* us reflects what is *inside* us. It's difficult to care about dolphins when we don't even care about ourselves. When we are sustained by impoverished hearts, when we feel that we can never get enough—of love, of food, or money—it is almost impossible to give. Love, food, money. A needy person impoverishes those around her. A vital person, on the other hand, lends vitality to those whom she touches. To be sensitive to the needs of the earth, we **must** be sensitive to our *own* needs. For when we feel the rapture of being alive, we feel tenderness towards all living things. And that is a tenderness our children cannot live without.

Index